PAIN PATTERNS

WHY YOU ARE IN PAIN AND HOW TO STOP IT

Rick Olderman MSPT

BOONE
PUBLISHING, LLC

Boone Publishing, LLC

Project Editor: Noah Charney
Book Cover Design: KÜCO Media
Interior Layout & Design: Urška Charney

Medical Illustrations:
Bence Berszán Árus
Martin Huber
Meghan Lewis

Boone Publishing, LLC www.BoonePublishing.com
Library of Congress Control Number: 2024913486

Library of Congress Subject Heading:

1. Backache—Physical Therapy—Treatment—Hand-books, manuals, etc. 2. Backache—Popular Works. 3. Back—Care & Hygiene—Popular Works. 4. Backache—Exercise Therapy. 5. Self-care, Health—Handbooks, manuals, etc. 6. Backache—Alternative Treatment. 7. Backache—Exercise Therapy. 8. Backache—Prevention. I. Title: Pain Patterns. Olderman, Rick. III. Title.

ISBN 978-0-9819152-1-0

Printed in the United States of America

Contents

This book is dedicated to those of you who are in pain and searching for solutions to your problem. I hope you find them here.

Preface

This workbook is for those of you with chronic back, sciatica or sacroiliac (SI) joint pain. These are the leading pain conditions that most people, including medical providers, struggle with. To me, this seems to indicate that we, in medicine, still have a lot to learn about these conditions. So, the good news is that the material here applies to chronic pain anywhere in the body, including hip, knee and neck pain, as well as migraines and headaches. My plan is simply for you to understand your specific body pain pattern and, in doing so, fix your pain.

My years as a physical therapist have led me to discoveries of pain patterns locked in place by muscle tension and movement habits. I introduced the idea of muscle tension in two of my earlier books, *Fixing You: Back & Sciatic Pain* (Boone Publishing, 2015) and *Solving the Pain Puzzle* (McFarland, 2023). However, I came to realize that these books gave many of you invaluable tools and materials to solve your pain but no clear blueprint to guide you. My intention is to remedy that with this workbook.

I am by no means a neuroscientist or here to walk you through a detailed neuroanatomical basis of movement. My goal is to simply help you understand why your body hurts and how to begin unraveling the mystery of why. It will involve learning a new way of thinking about your body—one that involves patterns of problems feeding your pain. To that end, I have included client stories throughout this book (while retaining total confidentiality and anonymity) to help illustrate these principles. While all the stories and details are true, I have changed names, genders, and merged details from other clients when one person's case hasn't included all the elements I discuss in that chapter. My hope is that this will more fully illuminate the principles laid out in these pages.

While the information in this book has solid medical research to support various facts, to my knowledge no one has assembled much of this information and thinking in one place, as I am now doing for you. My clinical successes and failures with my patients over the years are what have motivated me to integrate movement, fascia and neurological systems together into a treatment method. I am absolutely certain that many years from now, further improvements will occur by others who've taken up the torch but for now, this information presents a working understanding of why we have pain and how I have successfully managed to solve many difficult cases over the years.

I believe this book will help you understand, interpret, and simplify the pain messages you have been receiving. I think you will find the information and tests fascinating, fun, and revelatory. I hope to leave you with a solid plan to successfully fix your pain.

Introduction

Jim came to me with low-back and searing right-sided sciatic pain that erupted every time he bent down to sit or bent over to pick something up off the floor. Needless to say, he avoided these movements as much as he could. He was miserable. His pain was consistent and extreme, and he developed anxiety around anything linked to these behaviors.

After a thorough examination and full evaluation of the problem, I understood perfectly why this was happening.

"Jim, by the end of our session, you'll use bending down to fix your pain," I said.

He was surprised and very dubious that was possible.

What Jim did not understand was that the pain-producing movement simply revealed where and what the problem was. Jim used a pattern of movements to bend down and return upright that collectively caused his pain. Unfortunately, he was not aware of what these patterns were and why they were causing the problem.

By the end of our first session, and to Jim's delight, he could pick up a five-pound weight off the floor with no pain. In fact, doing so actually felt good. He simply changed his pattern of doing this simple activity which unloaded destructive forces from his back and pelvis.

This book represents my current understanding of movement patterns, often amplified by chronic tension, as a driver of chronic pain. I use the information you're about to read to help solve difficult pain problems. I hope it is a game-changer for you, as it has been for thousands of others.

Section 1   The Body's Language

This section lays out the three primary elements which weave together to create movement and, consequently, pain:

1. **Movement Habits**
2. **Fascial Networks**
3. **Reflex Patterns**

These three cords braid together to help us perform simple activities, such as standing up from a chair and walking across the room. How these simple tasks are performed, almost subconsciously, is influenced by our past history, lifestyle, and beliefs. At any given moment, we can become consciously aware of our actions. Therefore, we have all the tools necessary to transform any movement to solve pain—if only we understood what to focus on.

The first step, so to speak, is to gain a basic awareness of the roles of the above three elements. This knowledge is the language of the body. As with any language, once we have learned a few words, we can then begin to communicate.

Chapter 1   What is Chronic Pain?

Thirty years ago, at the beginning of my practice as a physical therapist, I came to the realization that the majority of my patients suffered from what is known as "chronic pain."

The term *chronic pain* refers to a timeline of pain that lasts for over three months during which time the body naturally heals. One of the first questions any medical provider will ask you when seeking help for your pain is, "How long have you been in pain?" We are trying to understand if this is an **acute** problem, meaning it has been going on for less than three months, or if it's a **chronic** problem, something that has lasted more than three months.

Usually within a three-month window, most damaged tissue will heal naturally, or at the very least be well on its way to healing, so that most pain will resolve on its own in that period. For example, a cut on your skin takes about 7-21 days to heal, a muscle strain or tear will take up to 2-3 months to mend depending on a few factors, and a fractured bone takes 6-8 weeks to knit together. For this reason, many treatments directed at solving back, sciatic or SI joint pain during this period are successful. If pain lasts beyond this three-month window, it is likely that something else is going on that is either prolonging the healing, re-irritating tissue, or referring pain from some other part or organ of your body.

Musculoskeletal pain can happen because of **viscerogenic** problems ("viscero" relates to organs and "-genic" refers to the origin). Viscerogenic pain is felt somewhere else in the body from where the source of the pain lies, usually in the musculoskeletal system, deriving from an organ-related issue.

The nerves that travel to and from our organs share the same intersections in our spine as the nerves that travel to and from our muscles. So, if an organ is in distress, it can send messages along its nerves which can at times become jumbled up with the nerve messages to and from our muscles. In these instances, our brain may sense back pain from an abdominal aortic aneurysm, kidney problem, or even a heart issue.

Various organs refer to different areas of the body—for instance heart, diaphragm and spleen issues can refer to the left shoulder or arm. Gallbladder or lung issues can refer to the right shoulder.[1] We medical providers are trained to be alert to and screen for these potential issues and refer patients to the appropriate medical professional for further testing if something seems amiss. However, in all my years in practice as a physical therapist, I cannot think of one case of chronic pain in my clinic that was due to viscerogenic issues. This is in large part due to our excellent doctors and physician assistants screening for these issues before a patient ever came to see me. Consequently, this guide will focus on chronic pain caused by non-viscerogenic issues found in joints, muscles or other musculoskeletal tissues.

> The term musculoskeletal collectively refers to our skeleton, fascia, muscles, ligaments, tendons and cartilage.

The International Association for the Study of Pain defines pain as: *"An unpleasant sensory and emotional experience associated with actual or potential tissue damage or described in terms of such damage."*[2] That "emotional experience" triggers our **autonomic nervous system (ANS)** which manages internal processes, including heart rate, blood pressure, respiration and digestion. The ANS is broken down into our **sympathetic nervous system (SNS)**—what is often referred to as the "fight or flight" nervous system—that helps us respond to threats or meet challenges, and the **parasympathetic nervous system (PSNS)**—our "rest and digest" nervous system—which calms our body back down after that threat or challenge is over. Personally, as a father, I have learned that the more I could help my children manage their emotional response to accidents, basically turning down their SNS response, the less pain they would "feel." Say my son fell and skinned his knee. If I reacted in a calm way, noting that this sort of thing happens all the time and it's nothing to worry about, then my son would shrug it off and move on, whereas if I made a big to-do over it, he would think he had really hurt himself, elevating his SNS response, and would be in more discomfort for longer.

Over the years as a physical therapist, I have come up with my own clinical definition of pain. It is simply: **An indication that something is wrong, right now**. Reframing pain as the body's way of alerting us to an immediate issue will create a subtle shift from seeing pain as an adversary to seeing it as a guide or teacher. This helped me discover and solve complex problems systematically and logically rather than simply trying to treat or soothe pain.

Take-Home Points

1. Pain often has an emotional component.

2. Our bodies heal quite well all by themselves within about three months of an injury.

3. Pain continuing after three months may be due to other complicating factors impeding or re-irritating tissues.

4. Re-framing your perspective to see pain as a signal that something is wrong at the moment, can lead to breakthroughs when solving chronic problems.

Chapter 2 Movement-Related Sources of Pain

As mentioned before, our body's internal systems can naturally heal most problems by themselves. In medicine, we rely heavily on this ability. By simply casting, bandaging, stitching up, or unloading those damaged tissues, your body can begin its natural mending process. At some point, most people will begin physical therapy to help restore length, strength, and function in order to return to their lifestyles.

If someone experiences pain after that mysterious three-month window, we then begin to suspect that something is impeding or blocking this healing process. In this situation, more tests are ordered, such as X-rays or an MRI, to reveal potential structural sources that were not considered before like arthritis, stenosis, tears, disc problems, etc. To date, we have no singular test, however, that identifies *why* tissues are damaged in chronic pain cases.

I have found that understanding *why* something is amiss is the key to truly solving chronic pain. Finding the "whys" requires a broader understanding of how you use all the parts of your body rather than simply the small area that experiences pain. In other words, helping you to solve the problem of chronic pain requires a **systems-thinking** approach.

Clinical Pearl

Research shows that, as we age, many types of change occur naturally and with increasing frequency in the spine.[3] Seeing disc degeneration (excessive wear and tear of the discs between the vertebrae) in a 20-year-old person has different implications than disc degeneration in an 80-year-old person. 37% of cases of disc degeneration in 20-year-olds were found to be asymptomatic (not causing pain), whereas 96% of cases involving disc degeneration in 80-year-olds were asymptomatic. In many cases, the older you are, the more likely it is that your orthopedist or primary care physician shrugs their shoulders with these types of findings and sends you to a physical therapist or other health care professional to figure out the real pain problem.

Physical therapists are musculoskeletal experts and have extensive medical training in how the muscles, tendons, ligaments, and bones are connected and how they influence each other. However, an orthopedic surgeon will have a greater understanding of specific tissues, such as intimate knowledge of how a rotator cuff muscle inserts at a specific point in the shoulder or about that tissue's integrity, but they may not fully understand how that shoulder is influenced by the position of the shoulder blade which is supported by the rib cage, which is affected by the pelvis, which responds to a myriad of other issues in the lower body system. That information does not make them better surgeons and that minutia of shoulder tissue detail will not necessarily help a physical therapist be better at their job, either. This is specialization in healthcare.

Dr. Shirley Sahrmann PT, PhD, FAPTA a physical therapist, professor, researcher, and clinician at Washington University in St. Louis, conducted extensive research, taught courses, and wrote textbooks about the intersection of movement and pain. As she states in her excellent textbook, *Diagnosis and Treatment of Movement Impairment Syndromes* (Mosby, 2002), "The loss of precise movement can begin a cycle of events that induces changes in tissues that progress from microtrauma to macrotrauma. Identification of the joint's directional susceptibility to movement (DSM) is the focus of the organization and naming of diagnostic categories."[4] Basically Dr. Sahrmann devised a system of categorizing movement impairments based on the movements that generated pain. Her work completely revolutionized my approach to solving chronic pain.

In terms of back pain, Dr. Sahrmann identified three *patterns* of movement impairments— Extension, Flexion and/or Rotation Problems— that underlie almost all spinal pain. [5]

Impairments are any irregularity of the anatomic, physiological, or psychological systems. Therefore, problems in any system or of any movement can contribute to musculoskeletal pain.[6]

Extension Problems

Extension Problems describe a spine that is either too arched (extended), undergoes too many forces trying to pull it into more of an arch, or lacks the structural integrity to resist those forces (Figure 2.1). Therefore, these types of problems would be characterized by spinal pain when the low back arches. Excessive arching of the lower spine contributes to increased compression on the **facet joints** (the bony parts of the vertebrae that contact the vertebra above or below).[7,8] People with an Extension Problem posture can be thought of as having a "military erect spine," one that is excessively or rigidly arched. Clinically, this is referred to as a lordotic posture, so named because of the excessive **lordosis** (arch in the lumbar spine) associated with this posture pattern. Often the pelvis is tilted forward (**anterior pelvic tilt**), accentuating the lumbar spine arch.

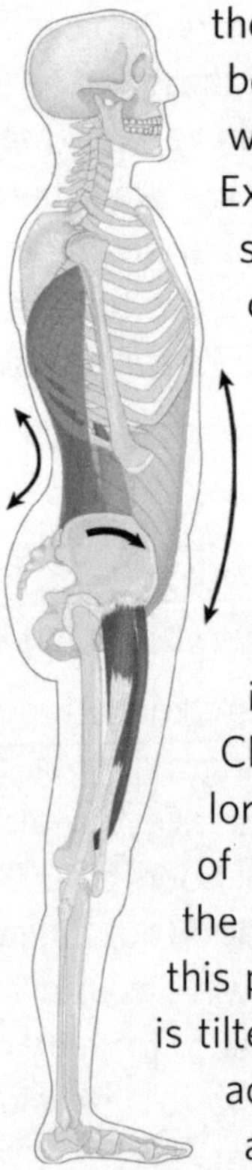

Figure 2.1 Extension Problems refer to back pain caused by either too much of an arch in the lower spine or too many forces trying to pull the spine into an arch.

Extension problems can occur when the lower back is excessively stiff and/or locked into an arched position, especially when bending over and returning to an upright position (Figure 2.2). This strategy is commonly taught in many ergonomic, fitness and exercise settings to protect the back. However, it often reinforces this pain pattern.

Clinically, I have found that Extension Problems cause more pain when *returning to an upright position from bending forward*, rather than bending forward itself. This places excessive strain on the junction between the pelvis and lumbar spine (see Chapter 3).

Lastly lordotic posture also occurs frequently during the later term of a pregnancy as a result of the fetus extending the belly while also adding weight to the front of the abdominal area (Figure 2.3). This pattern also occurs with people who are overweight and who carry much of that weight in their abdominal region.

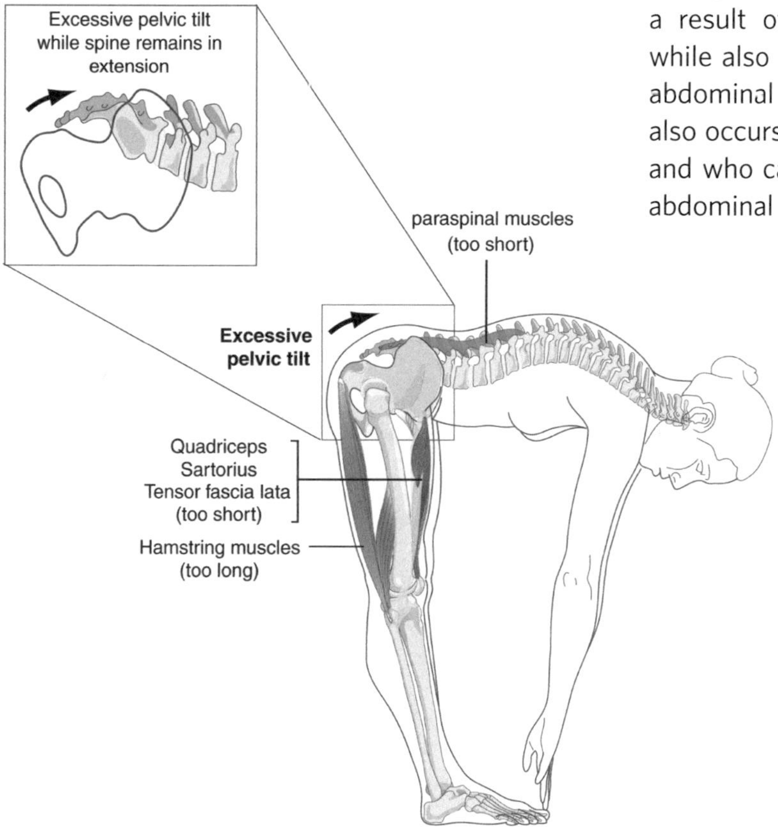

Excessive pelvic tilt while spine remains in extension

paraspinal muscles (too short)

Excessive pelvic tilt

Quadriceps
Sartorius
Tensor fascia lata
(too short)

Hamstring muscles
(too long)

Figure 2.2 Extension Problems are created when activating lower back muscles excessively and frequently during common activities such as bending forward.

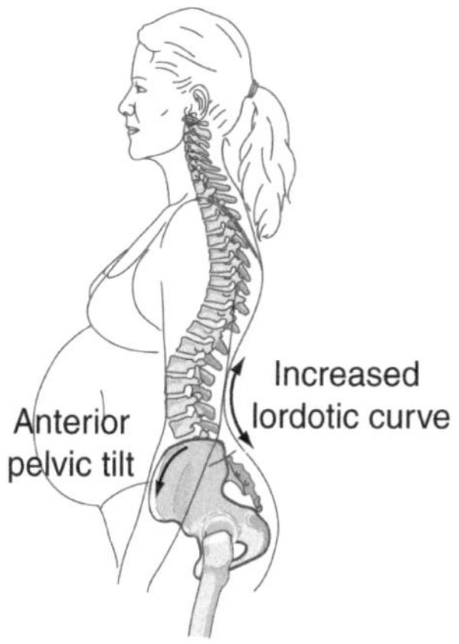

Increased lordotic curve

Anterior pelvic tilt

Figure 2.3 Later during pregnancy, growth of the fetus can contribute to excessive lordosis and therefore Extension Problems.

Flexion Problems

Flexion Problems describe a spine that is either too flat (flexed) or has the pull of too many flexion forces that are trying to flatten it (Figure 2.4). Basically, spinal pain would increase when the lower spine is flexed or flattened. This condition has been found to increase disc pressures between the vertebrae.[9,10]

Therefore more acute disc issues will be found in this population. Fortunately, these acute disc problems will often resolve on their own.[11] Flexion Problem postures often involve flat spines, excessive forces trying to flatten the spine or a lack of stability against those forces. Therefore, these are individuals who seem to slouch or lack an adequate lower spine arch. Often the pelvis is tilted backward (**posterior pelvic tilt**) contributing to the flatness of the spine.

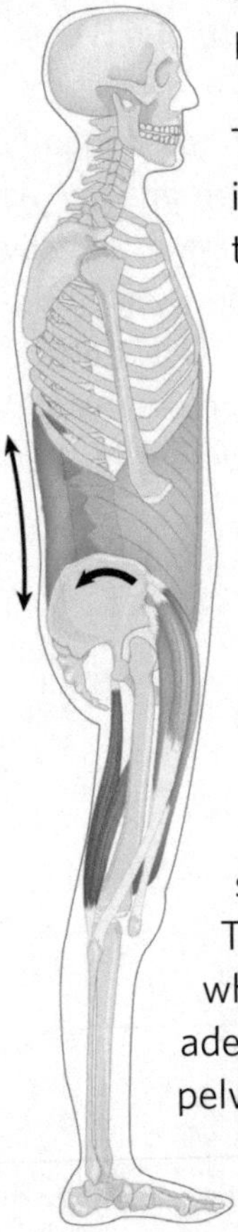

Flexion problems can occur when the lower back bends or flexes too soon, excessively or for too long when bending over and returning to an upright position (Figure 2.5).

Clinically, encountering this type of problem has been rare in my experience as in most cases the pain issue is spontaneously resolved without the need for any medical intervention.

Figure 2.4 Flexion Problems, the opposite of Extension Problems, refer to back pain caused by either too little arch in the lower spine or too many forces trying to flatten the spine.

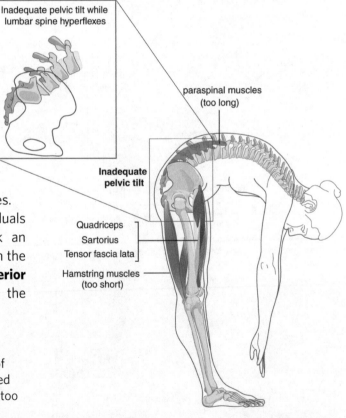

Inadequate pelvic tilt while lumbar spine hyperflexes

Inadequate pelvic tilt

paraspinal muscles (too long)

Quadriceps
Sartorius
Tensor fascia lata
Hamstring muscles (too short)

Figure 2.5 Flexion Problems are created when lower back muscles are excessively lengthened and remain so during common activities, such as bending forward.

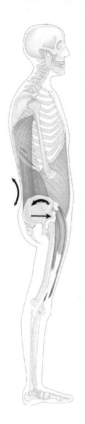

Swayback posture: this is one that involves the pelvic orientation of a Flexion Problem with the excessive arching of an Extension Problem (Figure 2.6), and can be thought of as a hybrid of these two patterns. This can be clinically difficult to diagnose, however the Extension/Flexion Test found in Chapter 6 will ultimately reveal the true pattern causing pain. Those of you with swayback posture test as Extension Problems, meaning your back feels better when slightly flatter than when arched, even though you may appear to have a Flexion Problem.

Figure 2.6 Swayback Posture involves components of both Extension and Flexion Postures.

I describe swayback posture as a "moping teenager" posture, where the upper body rests behind the pelvis and the pelvis is shifted forward when standing. Problems like these are more difficult to treat as well, however the Lifting the Rib Cage recommendation in Chapter 6, Butt Pumps in Chapter 10, and Gluteal or Tiptoe Walking in Chapter 11 are quite effective.

Rotation Problems

Rotation Problems describe a spine that is rotated in either direction (Figure 2.7). Dr. Sahrmann also includes sidebending movements with this category which I will discuss more in Chapter 4. Essentially, with these problems, rotating in the direction of the spinal rotation meets with less resistance or is less painful. In the figure below, right rotation would be easier and likely greater since her spine is right-rotated. Rotating in the opposite direction (left, if referring to the figure below) would be more restricted and likely painful.

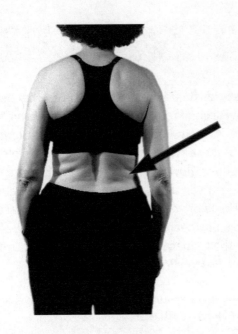

Figure 2.7 Rotation Problems involve vertebrae that are rotated. Note the right-side spinal muscles are larger than those on the left side. This is a consequence of vertebrae that are rotated to the right.

Rotation Problems can occur concurrently with Extension or Flexion Problems, and usually do. Therefore, solutions will simultaneously address both of these conditions.

Dr. Sahrmann referred to these dysfunctional patterns as **movement impairment syndromes**. In other words, these three larger patterns of problems describe the pain-producing strategies people use to create posture or when moving such as when bending over, sitting or walking. Repeating these strategies then creates vulnerabilities in the tissues undergoing the most movement. Typically, these areas experience more movement due to relative inflexibility or strength above and/or below that spinal section, which then overloads particular segments. This means that people create pain based on how they use their bodies—which makes intuitive sense. After all, movement is the one thing we all have in common.

Take-Home Points

1. Findings on scans take on different meanings as we age.

2. A systems understanding—one that identifies larger movement patterns that stress vulnerable tissues—helps solve chronic pain related to dysfunctional patterns.

3. There are three biomechanical patterns that contribute to most spinal pain as identified by Dr. Shirley Sahrmann: Extension Problems, Flexion Problems, and Rotation Problems. Rotation Problems can happen together with Extension or Flexion Problems.

Chapter 3 Fascia as a Source of Pain

My understanding of Dr. Sahrmann's information, while extremely helpful, did not address all chronic pain problems that I encountered at my clinic. There seemed to be connections in the body linking disparate regions together that functioned outside the scope of these three movement impairments. These connections seemed to involve **fascia.** Fascia is connective tissue that functions as a supporting and communicating network on a micro to macro level. Fascia invests in and blends with other tissues, like tendons, ligaments, and bone surfaces, often making it difficult to know where one tissue ends, and another begins. It also invests in and supports our organs, blood vessels and nerves. Fascia enables our body to do all the spectacular things we ask of it. Fascia is simply amazing!

In the human body, sometimes fascia is in the form of broad, tough sheaths, like the **iliotibial band (ITB)** on the side of the hip and upper leg (Figure 3.1), or **plantar fascia** on the bottom of the foot (Figure 3.2). In other areas, fascia exists in the form of webbing that holds small and large structures like blood vessels and nerves, in place. Essentially fascia is so deeply interwoven throughout the musculoskeletal system it would be difficult to find any example of movement or muscle contraction that doesn't involve fascia.

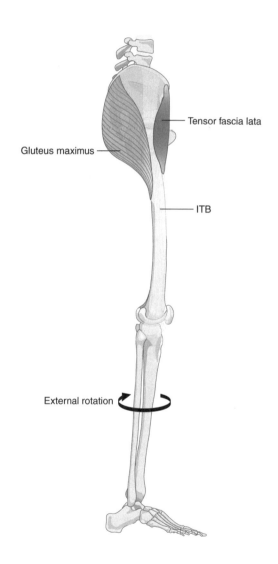

Figure 3.1 The iliotibial band (ITB) is fascia that connects the pelvis to the knee along the outside of the leg.

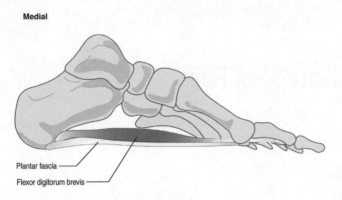

Medial

Plantar fascia
Flexor digitorum brevis

Figure 3.2 The plantar fascia connects the heel to the ball of the foot and supports the arch.

It is estimated that there are approximately 250 million nerves found in fascia.[12] Therefore fascia plays a significant role in sensing pain and, because fascia is literally everywhere in our body, it helps with our sense of **proprioception**— our understanding of where our body is in space at any given time—which is critical to postural and movement control. Like our muscles, bones and ligaments, the thickness and distribution of fascia constantly changes based on how we use our body.

Thomas Myers, manual therapist, fascial researcher and author of *Anatomy Trains: Myofascial Meridians for Manual and Movement Therapists, 4th edition* (Elsevier, 2021) identified what can be thought of as super-highways of fascia linking parts of the body together. In his fascinating book, he states, "Pattern recognition in posture and movement is a central skill to what we could call 'spatial medicine', the study of how we develop, how we stand, handle loads, move through our environment and occupy space—as well as how we perceive our bodily selves."[13] This highlights the importance of understanding and identifying pain patterns when solving difficult pain problems.

Because of fascia's significant networking connections, any part of the fascial web could influence a distant part of that system. This understanding helped me link possible pain culprits further from the site of pain. Here are a few of those fascial highways Mr. Myers identified (note that because fascia is so closely interconnected to muscles, tendons, and ligaments, it is easier to view fascial pathways by depicting those tissues as representations of fascia).

The Superficial Back Line

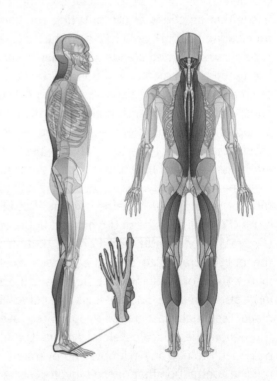

Figure 3.3 The Superficial Back Line of fascia ranges along the back of the body from the foot to the head.

The Superficial Front Line

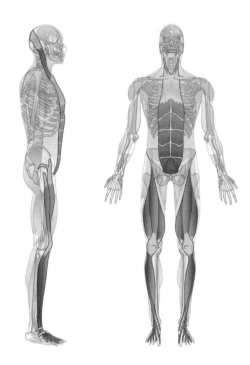

Figure 3.4 The Superficial Front Line of fascia extends along the front of the body.

The Spiral Line

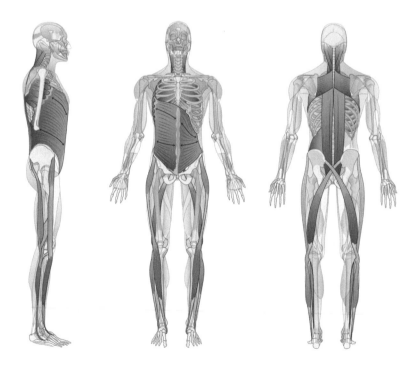

Figure 3.5 The Spiral Line of fascia spirals through the body. Note: the left external oblique and right internal oblique are not depicted in order to show the relationship between these two muscle/fascial groups.

The Lateral Line

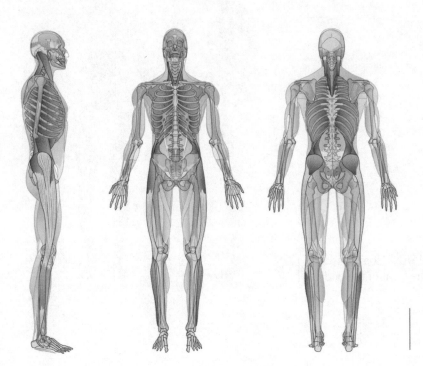

Figure 3.6 The Lateral Line of fascia exists along the sides of the body.

There is another line of fascia—the Deep Front Line (DFL)—that is a bit different from the others in that, according to Mr. Myers, "...there is no movement that is strictly the province of the DFL, yet neither is any movement outside its influence"[14] (Figure 3.7). Essentially I see the DFL as a significant deep supporter of the other lines of fascia and by extension, our structural integrity. Therefore, small deficiencies here will not play out immediately as a pain problem, but instead may be involved in more chronic issues.

As Mr. Myers puts it, "Thus many difficult-to-fix injuries are predisposed by an earlier failure within the DFL which is only revealed later when the precipitating incident takes place and exposes the core deficiency."[15] I would agree based on my clinical observations when helping people with difficult chronic pain problems. Typically, as I peel back layers of dysfunction in patients, elements of the DFL often need to be addressed.

The Deep Front Line

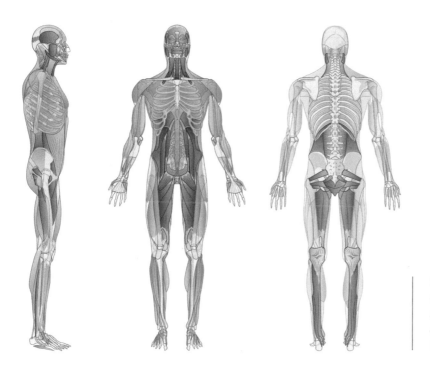

Figure 3.7 The Deep Front Line of fascia can be thought of as a deep supporter of other lines of fascia and our structural integrity.

Clinical Pearl

I have had success addressing the inner thigh muscles of the DFL using manual therapy techniques. Very often, there will be muscle fibers or zones that cause pain to be felt in (in medicine we say "refer to") the lumbar spine, SI joint or even the sciatic nerve down the same or opposite side of the body. I've even had cases where deep massage here has referred to the neck, head and even into the shoulder or down the arm. I believe in these cases I am affecting the connections of the DFL.

Section 2 of this book will help you identify the reasons these and other deep muscles develop painful points that refer to other areas of the body by unveiling larger movement patterns and asymmetries that ultimately affect this and other lines of fascia.

Visualizing these fascial highways, one can understand how foot dysfunction might be linked to head and neck pain, or pain anywhere in between. In fact, I once solved a woman's chronic headaches by treating her plantar fasciitis (foot pain).

Notice how the movement-based biomechanical patterns Dr. Sahrmann identified correspond very closely to the lines of fascia Thomas Myers articulated. When studying the images below, imagine the muscles along the fascial lines contracting and you can then see how that pattern would contribute to the associated movement patterns, or vice versa.

Extension Problems and the Superficial Back Line

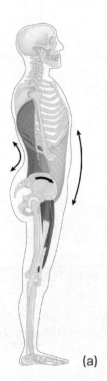
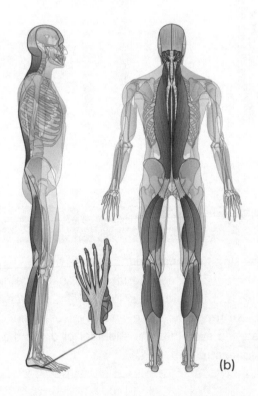

(a)

(b)

Figure 3.8 Extension Problems (a) involve the Superficial Back Line of fascia (b).

Flexion Problems and the Superficial Front Line and Deep Front Line

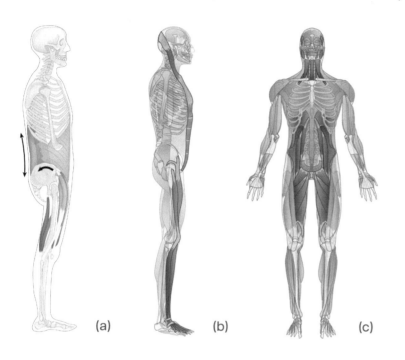

(a)   (b)   (c)

Figure 3.9 Flexion Problems (a) involve the Superficial Front Line (b) and/or Deep Front Line of fascia (c).

Rotation Problems and the Spiral Line

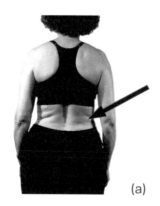

(a)

Figure 3.10 Rotation Problems (a) involve the Spiral Line of fascia (b) and the Lateral Line of fascia (c)—remember Dr. Sahrmann mentioned that Rotation Problems also involve lateral bending.

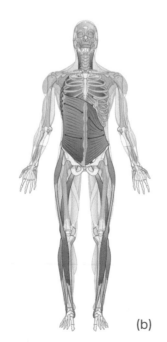

(b)

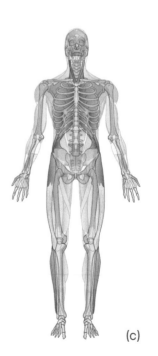

(c)

Myofibroblasts

Fascia is also invested with a type of **smooth muscle** which is different from skeletal muscle because it works on an involuntary basis (we cannot consciously make it contract).[16] Smooth muscle is mostly found in the organs of our gut and our blood vessels. Fascial smooth muscle is a little different because it responds to chemical stimulation rather than nerve stimulation that controls our skeletal muscles. More on this in just a moment.

Our fascial web is largely made up of a type of cell called **fibroblasts**. Fibroblasts are important in tissue repair—they aid scar formation and knit tissues together. A particular type of fibroblast, called **myofibroblasts**, has contractile properties similar to muscles ("myo-" refers to muscle). Myofibroblasts have up to six-times the contractile capacity of regular fibroblasts. While myofibroblasts may not exert a sufficient mechanical force to change immediate local biomechanics as a muscle could do, it seems they have a significant capacity to generate smaller forces sustained for longer periods of time. Interestingly, there is a higher concentration of myofibroblasts in the lower back region, in what is called the **thoracolumbar fascia**, than even the plantar fascia on the bottoms of our feet or the Iliotibial Band (ITB) on the sides of our legs.[17] The thoracolumbar fascia has a high concentration of both sensory (pain) and sympathetic nerve fibers meaning its nerves generate pain signals and are responsive to SNS output.[18]

Myofibroblasts are formed when regular fibroblasts undergo mechanical strain.[19] So if an area is not moving ideally or is subjected to repeated use or stress, myofibroblasts will develop in greater numbers in that region to support it.

Spinal Curves

Our spine has natural curves (Figure 3.11). Where those curves change direction, natural stress points are created. This means that mechanical stress is built into our spine even without adding any additional forces from muscles, fascia, or movement. Discs between the vertebrae of the spine help absorb and disperse this stress.

Figure 3.11 The spine has natural curves. Where curves change direction we find natural stress points buffered by spinal discs.

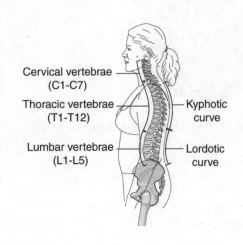

Cervical vertebrae (C1-C7)

Thoracic vertebrae (T1-T12)

Lumbar vertebrae (L1-L5)

Kyphotic curve

Lordotic curve

Most low back pain happens where the relatively smaller fifth lower back vertebra, **lumbar level five (L5)**, meets with the relatively larger pelvis by interacting with the **sacrum (S1)**, a triangle-shaped bone in the pelvis which is composed of fused vertebrae. Notice that the sacrum is also curved and so the junction of the sacrum and lumbar spine represents yet another change in curve direction and another potential mechanical stress point along the spine.

The sacrum is sandwiched between two large bones called **ilia**, which house the hip sockets with which the thigh bones (**femurs**) articulate to form the hip joints. The **pelvis** is composed of these three bones and, along with the lumbar spine, they form the biomechanical center of the body (Figure 3.12).

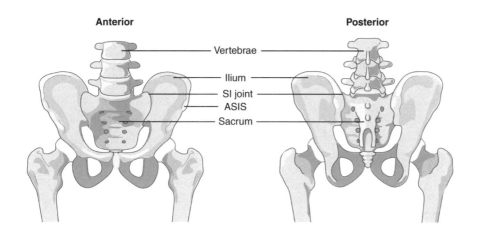

Figure 3.12 The pelvis comprises three bones: two ilia and one sacrum. The sacrum (S1) articulates with the lowest lumbar vertebra (L5).

The pelvis is large and basically moves as one unit. Very large muscle groups like the **quadriceps** (in the front of the thigh), **hamstrings** (in the back of the thigh), **adductors** (along the inner thigh) or **gluteal** (butt or rear-end) muscles attach to the pelvis from the legs. These muscles are relatively long and powerful and consequently exert significant mechanical force to the pelvis. Sometimes those forces are balanced and symmetrical and sometimes those forces are unbalanced and asymmetrical.

To envision how the leg muscles might affect the pelvis and spine, imagine trying to move a large boulder. It is much easier to move that boulder if you use a lever. The longer the lever arm, the more dramatic its impact on the boulder. To put it simply, this is how the legs generate significant force and tension to the pelvis and, by extension, the spine—they apply leverage force to the pelvis.

The lumbar vertebrae are smaller and more mobile relative to the larger pelvis (Figure 3.13), to which they must react. Where the sacrum (S1) meets the lowest lumbar vertebra (L5), the greatest mechanical stress will affect the spine due to this inequity in size, mobility, and change in curve direction. This makes intuitive sense— things that move more (the L5/S1 junction) have a higher likelihood of breaking down than things that don't move (the pelvis).

The junction between these two areas will most likely be the area of the most dramatic stress, tissue damage, and thus pain. This explains why there seems to be a higher rate of degenerative changes in the lumbar spine involving L5/SI pathology rather than L1/L2 (lumbar vertebrae higher up in the spine).[20]

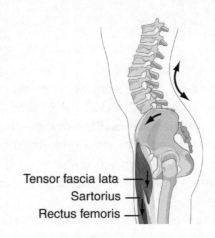

Tensor fascia lata
Sartorius
Rectus femoris

Figure 3.13 Large muscles from the legs attach to and affect the pelvis which in turn affect the spine.

This may also explain why there is a high concentration of myofibroblasts (contracting fibroblast cells) in the lumbar region—to help stabilize this zone of mechanical stress.

Transforming Growth Factor βeta 1

Unlike regular muscle that responds to nerve signals, myofibroblasts respond to a hormone-like molecule called a **cytokine**, specifically transforming growth factor βeta 1 (TGF β1).[21,22] TGF-β1 levels can increase due to an immune response from the SNS.[23,24,25] The SNS typically activates in stressful situations, such as when we are threatened, in danger, experience physical or emotional trauma, or are under continuous pressure.[26] So ultimately, SNS stimulation can lead to fascial tension along the superhighways identified by Thomas Myers, or more specifically in areas of mechanical stress where myofibroblasts have formed.

It appears that myofibroblasts do not contract like muscles. Typically, when a muscle receives a signal along a nerve to contract, it happens very quickly and is sustained until that signal is turned off again. Think about bending your elbow. Your biceps muscles on the front of your upper arm receive a message from your brain to contract. Then those muscles relax once that message is turned off.

While muscles may directly affect joint or postural mechanics, myofibroblasts seem to have a prolonged and perhaps subtler effect. Because myofibroblasts respond to TGF-β1 levels, their contraction ramps up and down much more slowly, creating a relatively sustained low-grade contraction for minutes and perhaps many hours.[27] This may have a profound effect on lumbopelvic dynamics. Since muscles respond to nerve signals from the brain but myofibroblasts respond to TGF-β1 circulating in our system, those TGF-β1 levels may remain elevated even after the brain has turned off signals to the muscles in that region. This can then contribute to chronic tension in that region.

This may be how emotional or psychological events manifest as back pain—because of the high concentration and activation of myofibroblasts in that region from elevated TGF-β1 concentrations. Especially when considering cases of post-traumatic stress disorder (PTSD), chronic anxiety, or deep-seated trauma, the SNS is often re-activated again and again, potentially creating a steady release of TGF-β1 which then activates myofibroblasts contributing to chronic tension in whatever zones those myofibroblasts are inhabiting. Likewise, other areas of mechanical strain in the body may develop a higher concentration of myofibroblasts, creating an environment for emotional trauma to be lodged in those zones of mechanical stress as well.

Take-Home Points

1. Fascia connects everything in our bodies. There are superhighways of fascia linking the feet to the head along different lines in the body that closely correspond to Dr. Sahrmann's movement impairment patterns.

2. Myofibroblasts, which have up to six times the contractile capacity of regular fascia, are laid down in mechanically stressed areas of our bodies, such as the low back.

3. Myofibroblasts can be activated to contract when the fight-or-flight nervous system, the SNS, is triggered and sustains longer periods of contraction when compared to muscle stimulation via nerves.

Chapter 4   Your Brain and Body Connection

Understanding fascia has taught me that the *site* of pain might not actually be the *source* of the pain. After realizing the connection between movement patterns, fascia, and the SNS, I needed to better under-stand these pathways, which meant learning more about the **brain**.

Our brains are designed for success. If your goal is to get from A to B, your brain will figure out the best way to achieve that goal. If that effort is repeated often, your brain will create greater efficiency to complete that task, which is the purpose of practice. As far as chronic pain is concerned, it seems the brain is primarily concerned with *your short-term plan of* achieving that goal and will subtly negotiate obstacles along its path to achieve immediate success. However with regards to the body, these short-term adaptations can lead to subconscious compensations that break down our body's tissues over time.

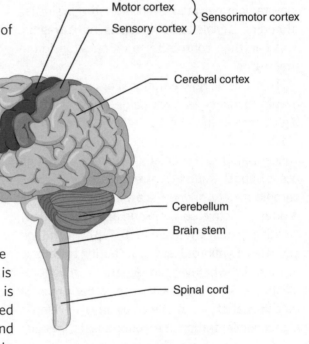

Motor cortex
Sensory cortex
} Sensorimotor cortex

Cerebral cortex

Cerebellum

Brain stem

Spinal cord

Figure 4.1 The brain. The cerebral cortex is the outer layer of the brain, composed of many folds.

The Brain & Spinal Cord

All muscles in some way report and respond to the brain via nerves, and so the ultimate control of movement and muscle tension is found in our brain (Figure 4.1).

There are two areas of the brain that I will focus on in this regard: the cerebral cortex and the cerebellum.

1. The **cerebral cortex**, our most evolu-tionarily advanced area, is responsible for higher executive functioning and contains, among other structures, the sensory and motor cortices (plural for cortex) from which conscious sensation, such as touch, occurs and movement is initiated.

Looking at Figure 4.1, you will see two zones in the middle of the cerebral cortex, one for the **motor cortex** and one for the **sensory cortex** (together these are referred to as the **sensorimotor cortex**). The motor cortex is primarily devoted to control of our muscles and movement patterns and the sensory cortex receives information about what's happening with our body. Together they help us coordinate movement and respond to environmental concerns.

Embedded in the sensorimotor cortex is a map of our body, called a **homunculus** (Figure 4.2). The body is depicted on this map according to the importance of the structure in question.

For example, the hands, face, and feet are very important to us for manipulating objects, communication, and locomotion and so our motor cortex map has a larger percentage of space devoted to these three important functions. Sensory information, like touch or pain from the body, is similarly mapped in the sensory cortex. A recent study has shown that, with regards to the motor cortex, the homunculus map can change with training.[28] Therefore changing how you use your body to create better, less painful strategies for movement will also change your brain, to reinforce those strategies.

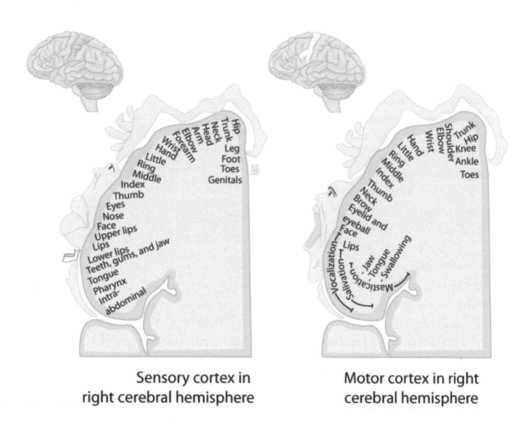

Sensory cortex in
right cerebral hemisphere

Motor cortex in right
cerebral hemisphere

Figure 4.2 Homunculi of the sensory and motor cortices represent relative functional importance as it is mapped in the brain.

2.   The second area is the **cerebellum** which is located behind the brainstem and below the cerebral cortex (see Figure 4.1). This area is responsible for coordination, storing, and retrieving habitual patterns of movement, such as sitting down, typing on a computer, working on an assembly line or walking. It is also important in maintaining muscle tone and helps with postural control.

Extending further down are the **brainstem** and **spinal cord** (see Figure 4.1), which house **nerve tracts**—specialized highways running to and from the brain and body. These tracts are dedicated solely to carrying certain types of information.

For example, the **corticospinal tract** is a motor tract that communicates messages directly to muscles, instructing them to relax or contract in varying degrees. This descending tract is a one-way street extending from the motor cortex of our brain down the spinal cord, which then communicates with a nerve that connects to a muscle (Figure 4.3).

There is also the **spinocerebellar tract**, which carries subconscious sensory information in the opposite direction, to the cerebellum (Figure 4.3). This tract helps us with posture, coordinating movements, muscle tone, and understanding where our limbs are in space (proprioception). This is a sensory tract because it runs up to the brain from our body.

Finally, I should mention the **dorsal columns/ medial lemniscus (DCML) pathway** (Figure 4.3). This tract carries similar information to the spinocerebellar tract, except that this is information we are *consciously* aware of, such as fine or discriminating touch or vibration or our sense of proprioception. This tract goes to our sensory cortex, rather than the cerebellum.[29]

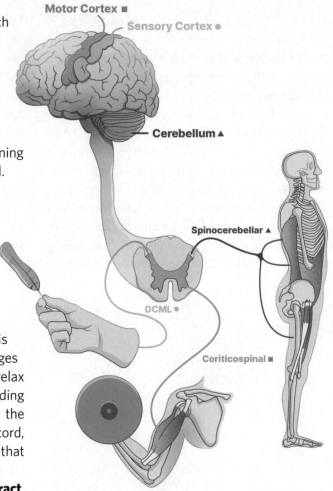

Figure 4.3 The corticospinal, spinocerebellar, and dorsal columns/medial lemniscus (DCML) tracts carry information to and from our body to help our brain negotiate our environment.

Both the brain and the spinal cord comprise the **central nervous system (CNS)**. Nerves that exit or enter the spinal cord to and from our muscles are called **peripheral nerves** and are part of the **peripheral nervous system** (**PNS**), because they travel to our periphery—muscles, tendons, ligaments etc. The brain then coordinates movement via these and other tracts running through our spinal cord to and from our body.

> **Clinical Pearl**
>
> Peripheral nerves leaving the lumbar spine and sacrum bundle together to form the large **sciatic nerve** which feeds the lower body muscles. This also occurs in the upper body system, however the nerves blend to form three larger nerves: **radial**, **ulnar**, and **median**. Radiating nerve pain, **radicular** or **radiculopathy pain**, involves irritation of these peripheral nerves. There are many reasons why someone may experience radiculopathy. Medical providers focus primarily on the spine structures or disease processes as the causes of radiculopathy. However this book will help you see that is only part of the picture in many cases.

Muscle Spindles, Proprioception & Reflexes

Embedded in our muscles are small, complicated structures called **muscle spindles** which are sensitive to the change in velocity of lengthening muscles. They communicate with, and are monitored by, our brain to help our muscles adapt to changes in the length of those muscles.[30]

Muscle spindles are a type of **mechanoreceptor**—a structure that alerts us to changes in stretch, shear, compression, force, etc. There are many types of mechanoreceptors that are specialized according to the different types of forces they monitor. They include: free nerve endings, Ruffini corpuscles, lamellated corpuscles, and Golgi tendon organs.

Mechanoreceptors exist in fascia and muscle and the information they gather and transmit to the brain, together with the complicated fascial connections to, in and through our muscles, help us to understand where and how we are in space. In other words, mechanoreceptors help us with proprioception and therefore movement and postural control.

Returning our attention to muscle spindles, remember that fascia is deeply integrated into muscle cells and bands of muscle fibers. It has been shown that muscle spindles' outer capsules are continuous with fascia that surround each muscle.[31] [32]

One of the muscle spindles' primary roles is to help protect muscle by signaling them to contract when excessive or rapid lengthening occurs. We learned in Chapter 3 that fascia is closely interwoven into the musculoskeletal system. Therefore, muscle spindle activity not only applies to muscles but also extends to our fascia network potentially affecting those structures near or far, directly or indirectly. Hopefully you will now be gaining an appreciation for the complexity of sensing and creating movement which has traditionally been ascribed only to muscles, but which we now understand has just as much to do with our fascial network.

Perhaps the most popular example of muscle spindle activity is the **knee-jerk reflex** (Figure 4.4). When the knee is bent and the knee tendon is tapped with a small reflex hammer (causing a rapid lengthening of that muscle/tendon complex), the thigh muscle then immediately contracts, kicking the foot up into the air. This

stretch reflex response happens without conscious involvement and helps protect the thigh muscle from becoming damaged. The brain is alerted milliseconds after the reflex has actually occurred. This reflexive communication between the brain, muscles and spindles is a primary way our muscle, and likely fascia, tone or tension is maintained.

Too little a kick during the knee-jerk reflex could indicate a potential PNS problem—a disruption in the nerve pathway leading to the muscle from the spine. Essentially, the muscle is unable to receive a sufficiently strong signal to contract. This is why it is important to try to obtain an accurate response to this simple test—it gives us foundational information about the integrity of our nervous system.

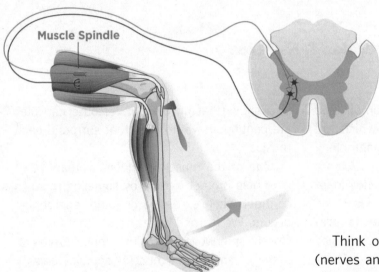

Muscle Spindle

Figure 4.4 The knee-jerk reflex occurs via the muscle spindle communicating a rapid change in muscle length.

Clinically, we use the knee-jerk test to glimpse the integrity of the nervous system. An abnormally strong knee-jerk response can indicate a problem in the CNS (the brain or spinal cord), such as in a stroke victim or someone with a traumatic brain injury. If there is a disruption in the CNS feedback system between the brain and the body, the brain cannot down-regulate muscle contraction which can result in muscle rigidity or spasm.

Think of muscle tone as a **neuromuscular** (nerves and the muscles they invest in) state of readiness. People who exercise often have greater muscle tone in part because their neuromuscular system is frequently challenged, and so it maintains this state of readiness in the form of a small, unconscious amount of muscular stimulation of frequently recruited muscles. Muscle **tension** also involves muscle tone. However, in this book I use this term to denote tone that results in excessive tissue strain or pain. Ultimately muscle tone and tension involve the complex interplay of our brain, muscle spindles, nervous system, muscles and fascia.

Large Reflex Patterns

Unlike the simple knee-jerk reflex, there are more expansive reflexes which involve multiple muscle groups over several joints throughout the body. In other words, they involve *patterns of movement*. These are hardwired into our nervous system as we develop in the womb. They are the Startle, Landau and Withdrawal/Crossed Extensor Reflexes.

Startle Reflex

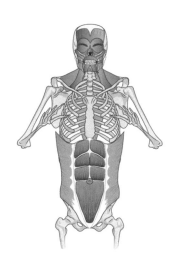

The **Startle Reflex** can be triggered by all five senses but usually by sudden, loud noises or some other noxious stimuli or stressor. The most common contraction pattern for this reflex is for the eyes to blink, shoulders to lift, neck muscles to contract and arms to flex (Figure 4.5). This reflex helps us protect our head, neck, and organs from danger by causing us to fold forward and retract our head like a turtle. Abdominal contractions have also been noted with this reflex pattern.[33]

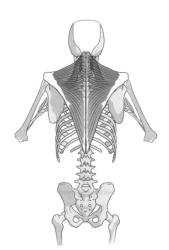

Figure 4.5 The Startle Reflex includes facial, shoulder, and abdominal contraction patterns.

Landau Reflex

The **Landau Reflex** helps our nervous system develop while we are still in the womb. We first use this reflex after a few months of age, to lift our head and arch the spine in order to crawl. Thomas Myers touches on this briefly in *Anatomy Trains: Myofascial Meridians for Manual Therapists & Movement Professionals* (Elsevier, 2021) stating, "In human development, the muscles of the SBL [Superficial Back Line of fascia], lift the baby's head from embryological flexion, with progressive engagement and 'reaching out' through the eyes, supported by the SBL."

As we grow, this reflex is somewhat overridden by common daily activities. However, when we need to respond to a stressful situation, we tap into this ancient reflex pattern, triggering contraction along the spine to bring us to an erect, ready posture (Figure 4.6).[34] This helps us see and respond to the threat.

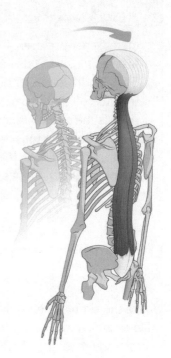

Figure 4.6 The Landau Reflex includes muscles that help extend our neck and back.

Withdrawal Reflex/Crossed Extensor Reflex

The third pattern is the **Withdrawal Reflex**. In the upper body, this involves triggering the upper body flexor muscles (muscles that bend joints) to withdraw from a painful stimulus, like pulling your hand away after touching a hot stove. In the lower body, this phenomenon involves activating the **Crossed Extensor Reflex**. Again, the limb that has come into contact with something painful withdraws by contracting the lower body and waist muscles on that side but which also causes the opposite leg muscles to straighten (extend) the stance leg, so we don't fall down at the same time (Figure 4.7).

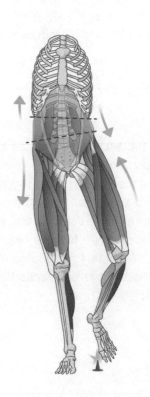

Figure 4.7 The Crossed Extensor Reflex activates flexion (bending) contraction of muscles on one side of the lower body while extending (straightening) the limb of the opposite side to prevent falls.

To get a clear picture of the Crossed Extensor Reflex, imagine stepping on a nail with your left foot. The pain immediately triggers the left pelvis and leg to withdraw. But to do that safely, the right leg needs to hold you up just as quickly. The left knee, hip and waist muscles will contract to remove weight off that nail. Because the waist muscles also connect to the ribcage, it is not uncommon to find one side of the rib cage sitting lower than the other because of chronic engagement of this pattern (Figure 4.7). Because this pattern involves an uneven pelvis, it is commonly misdiagnosed as a **leg-length discrepancy**—a difference in the length of the legs.

Clinical Pearl

Many people are given a diagnosis of a leg-length discrepancy when their practitioner notices that one side of the pelvis is higher or lower than the other when standing. However, this does not consider the tension and compensations that occur through multiple joints in the lower body and pelvic system to create this postural illusion. Clinically I have found leg-length discrepancies quite rare when the actual thigh and lower leg bones are measured.

According to Dr. Thomas Hanna, the developer of *Hanna Somatics*, all three reflex patterns (Startle, Landau, and Withdrawal/Crossed Extensor) can be found to some extent in any individual. The presence of these patterns is attributed to the fact that the brain and body (or **soma**—hence *Soma*tics) have forgotten how to move out of them (established cerebellar pathways) and are heavily influenced by their existence. Dr. Hanna refers to this motor forgetfulness as **sensory motor amnesia (SMA)**, which is actually a cerebellar/sensorimotor cortex/muscle spindle pathway problem.

Interestingly, in his book, *Fascia: The Tensional Network of the Human Body* (Elsevier, 2022), Dr. Robert Schleip, a fascia researcher and manual therapist, relates a story whereby two conflicting schools of thought approached the idea of movement restrictions, tension or resistance to movement differently. One ascribed restrictions to a brain-based phenomena and the other ascribed it to purely mechanical fascial adhesions or restrictions. Dr. Schleip created a small experiment whereby three subjects' passive range of motion was measured, then they were given a general anesthetic during which their passive range of motion was re-measured and found to be significantly greater. This little experiment helped show that, in this case anyway, movement restrictions had less to do with mechanical shortness of tissues and more to do with neurological input and output from the CNS and PNS.[35]

This helps support Dr. Hanna's assertions that the reason muscles along these reflex patterns do not lengthen smoothly—instead exhibiting a type of holding pattern—is a result of subconscious muscular tension coupled with an inability to inhibit those contractions efficiently and smoothly. Central to all three reflex patterns (as well as their related fascial and movement patterns) are the muscles involved in the lumbopelvic region, which is the body's center of function and the site of most fundamental changes in the musculoskeletal system in response to movement dysfunction, emotional stress, or trauma. When subconscious tension occurs in this "somatic center," a ripple of compensations can extend to other muscles and joints throughout the kinetic chain (Figure 4.8).

These compensatory changes can occur from the bottom up (as in the case of a painful foot stepping on a nail creating a Crossed Extensor Reflex response) or top down (as in the case of a sciatica causing numbness or weakness in the lower body, therefore causing peripheral problems that then likely biomechanically feed back up to the pelvis). I discuss this in more detail in Chapter 5.

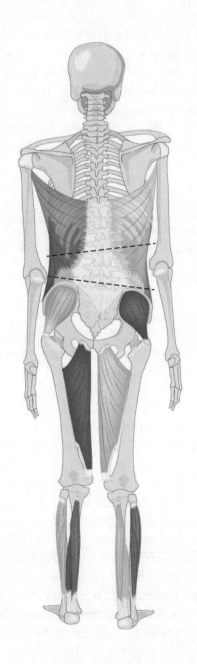

Figure 4.8 Ripple effects occur throughout the body in response to movement, fascial- and reflex-related changes.

Putting It All Together

Notice that these three reflex patterns match almost perfectly with the fascial superhighways discovered by Thomas Myers and the biomechanical movement impairment dysfunction patterns discovered by Dr. Shirley Sahrmann.

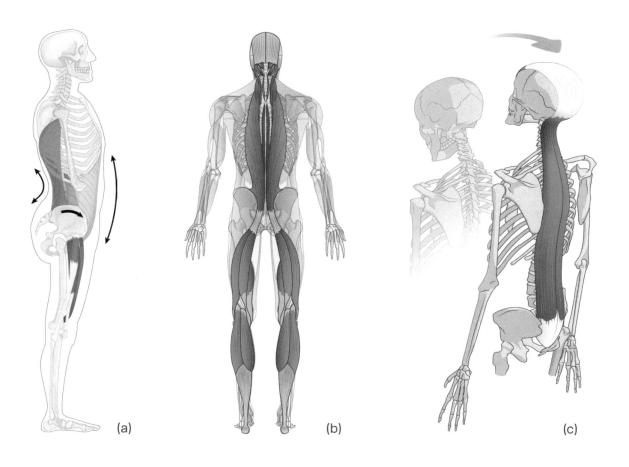

(a)   (b)   (c)

Figure 4.9 Extension Problems (a) and the Back Line pattern of fascia (b) correspond to the Landau Reflex pattern of contraction (c) in which the back muscles contract to bring us into an alert posture.

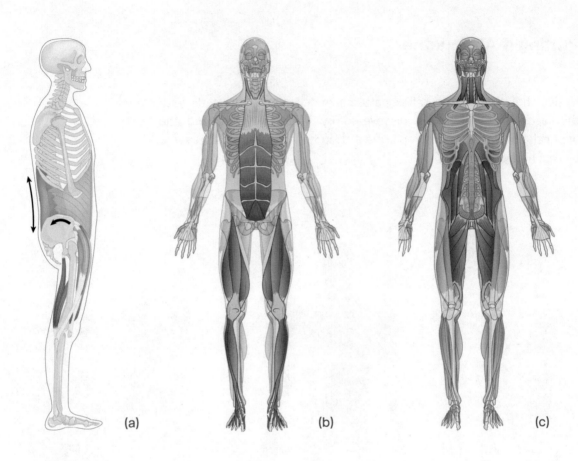

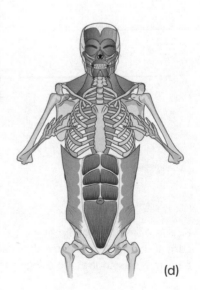

Figure 4.10 Flexion Problems (a) and the Front Line pattern of fascia (b) as well as the Deep Front Line of fascial pattern (c) correspond to the Startle Reflex pattern of contraction (d) in which the muscles in the front of the trunk contract to bring us into a protective posture.

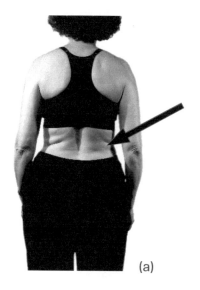

(a)

Figure 4.11 Rotation Problems (a) and the Lateral and Spiral Line patterns of fascia (b & c) correspond to the Withdrawal/Crossed Extensor Reflex pattern of contraction (d) in which the waist and pelvic muscles contract to unload a unilateral injury to our lower body.

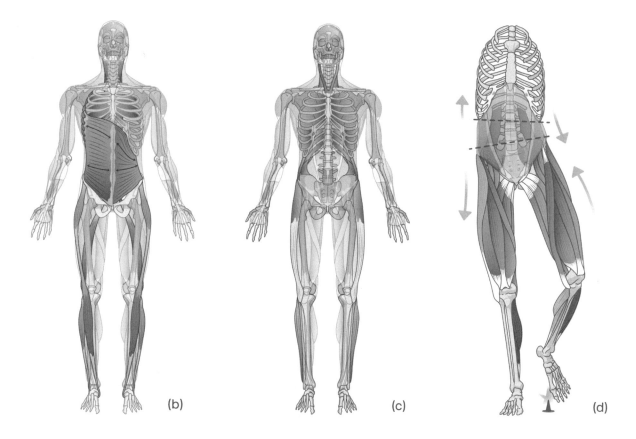

(b)   (c)   (d)

The one disparity is that Dr. Sahrmann's third pattern is a Rotation Problem (which she states includes lateral bending) but the Withdrawal/Crossed Extensor Reflex is a lateral (side) pattern. Remember that Thomas Myers identified both lateral *and* spiral lines of fascial superhighways. This apparent inconsistency is explained by Fryette's Laws, developed back in 1918 by the osteopath Harrison Fryette. Fryette's first law states that when the spine is in a neutral orientation, such as when standing upright, *lateral sidebending (a term I've coined to describe this phenomenon) creates opposite-side rotation*. This means the lateral versus rotation discrepancy is really the same problem with two different perspectives, like light being both a particle and a wave. Because lateral sidebending drives rotation to the opposite side, it is accurate to refer to this pattern more simply as a **Sidebending Problem**, the hallmarks of which are an uneven pelvis and rib cage (elements of a Crossed Extensor Reflex pattern).

Viewing the image of a Rotation Problem from Chapter 2, now pay attention to the larger crease in the left waist muscles—a sign of a Sidebending Problem due to an uneven pelvis and rib cage (Figure 4.12). The thick spinal muscles indicating the right-rotated vertebrae identified earlier are actually *responding to* the Left Sidebending Problem which creates the rotated vertebrae.

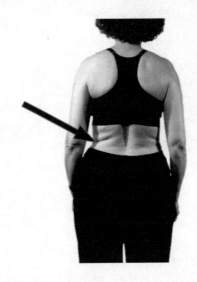

Figure 4.12 The larger left waist crease indicates a Left Sidebending Problem which drives right-rotation of the vertebrae. Looking closely, one can see the patient's left side of her pelvis is higher than the right side indicating a Sidebending Problem.

Naming the patterns of problems regardless of the tissues or responses that are creating them keeps this pattern identification simple and straightforward:

Extension Problems are those where the spine is too arched (extended) or where there are too many forces trying to pull it into an arch.
Flexion Problems are those where the spine is too flat (flexed) or there are too many forces trying to reduce its arch.
Sidebending Problems are those where the pelvis is higher on one side and the rib cage is lower, usually on that same side. The Sidebending Problem is named for the side where this is happening. So, Figure 4.12 depicts a Left Sidebending Problem. If the pelvis is higher on one side and the rib cage is lower on the opposite side, then that is referred to as a **Complex Sidebending Problem**, discussed more in Chapter 7.

Extension Problems or Flexion Problems can happen together with Sidebending Problems and usually do, especially in cases of one-sided back pain, sciatica (usually felt in one leg) or SI joint pain. Of course, Extension Problems and Flexion Problems typically do not happen concurrently because they are opposing patterns (although I mention a caveat to this general rule in Chapter 6). You will test for these problems in Chapters 6 and 7.

In my clinical experience, chronic pain cases usually involve muscle tension corresponding to these three movement, fascial, and reflexive patterns. Many treatments for back, sciatica, or SI joint pain involve a small zone of treatment—usually in the immediate area of pain. This is often why chronic pain exists—the larger pain patterns of dysfunction have not been considered or addressed, and so pain often returns. These patterns exert significant leverage and force to injured or damaged tissues, causing pain and/or physical changes in the tissues. As Dr. Sahrmann puts it, "The loss of precise movement can begin a cycle of events that induces changes in tissues that progress from micro-trauma to macrotrauma."[36]

Section 2 of this book contains several tests to determine the existence of these patterns and some of their root causes, as well as exercises or habit modifications to eliminate them. This should significantly reduce chronic pain.

Take-Home Points

1. Muscle tone/tension, postural control and movement are achieved through a complex interplay of many components of our musculoskeletal and nervous systems.

2. Older, hardwired reflex patterns closely align with both fascial superhighways and movement dysfunction patterns described in Chapters 2 and 3. They are: Startle Reflex, Landau Reflex, Withdrawal/Crossed Extensor Reflex.

3. Combining these three sources of dysfunction (movement, fascial, reflexive) these patterns are more simply identified as: Extension Problems, Flexion Problems, Sidebending Problems.

4. Sidebending Problems can and often do occur together with Extension or Flexion Problems and are usually involved in one-sided back, sciatic, or SI joint pain.

Chapter 5   Functional Linking

Client Connection

I recently worked with a woman over a Zoom video call and who developed left-sided sciatic pain after a particular exercise she performed in her CrossFit class. Her pain remained constant through several types of treatments over many months. Within a few minutes of working with her, we identified Extension and Sidebending Problems as her pain patterns. Taking her through the tests in Section 2 of this book, we uncovered several older, pre-existing problems of which she was unaware. Only after addressing those hidden issues that fed her Sidebending and Extension Problems did her pain completely melt away. While the CrossFit exercise was a trigger for her pain, the causes were found in older, deeper, hidden problems.

To understand how the three pain patterns we have discussed cause tension and pain, remember how they began in the first place. Long ago, habits were adopted in response to lifestyle, injuries, sports, work, psychological stressors, etc. Repeated behaviors like weight-bearing on one leg more than the other, maintaining an excessively stiff back when bending over, faulty walking patterns or simply habitually sitting at an angle to work may have created ripple effects throughout the body. As Dr. Sahrmann puts it, "...causes of deviations in joint movement patterns are *repeated movements* and *sustained postures* associated with daily activities of work and recreation."[37]

Because your brain is wired for short-term success, it creates alternative movement patterns—compensations—for problems that arise. This taps into the biomechanical movement patterns explored in Chapter 2 which coincide with the fascial superhighways running through our bodies discussed in Chapter 3 and are reinforced by the hardwired reflex patterns mentioned in Chapter 4 that extend across multiple muscles and joints.

The cerebellum, working with the motor and sensory cortices of the cerebral cortex, reinforces these neural pathways so these habitual movements can be accessed and carried out faster and automatically. This results in overuse issues for those parts of the body that carry more of the burden and contributes to rigidity in the muscles, fascia, ligaments, or tendons that are involved in these patterns. This rigidity is maintained in part through muscle spindle adaptations, sensitizing muscles to changes in length, which helps create a state of readiness in the form of muscle tone or tension for these frequently used muscles in these commonly used patterns.

These frequent movement patterns tend to break down or slowly degrade the joints, and their associated tissues housed within their patterns which move more or are more susceptible to stress. This creates inflammation and signals the body to lay down myofibroblasts to reinforce that area of mechanical strain. Myofibroblasts, susceptible to SNS activation from emotional trauma, anxiety, or stress potentially add prolonged fascial contraction to a mechanically stressed area of the body. The body tries to play catch-up to repair the daily damage these overuse patterns create, but it can never repair the damage fast or completely enough. This is when chronic pain emerges.

> Wolff's Law in medicine states that our bones respond to forces acting on them over time, becoming thicker or thinner. For instance, habitually increasing load to a bone can increase its thickness,[38] whereas prolonged unloading of bone, such as during bed rest, can lead to bone loss.[39] Davis's Law is like Wolff's Law, however it applies to soft tissues, like muscle or tendon. An example of this would be the loss of sarcomeres (the smallest functional unit of a muscle) in the calf muscles as a result of wearing high heels.[40] Therefore, our bodies are constantly responding and adapting to stresses, both physical and mental.[41]

Compensation Patterns and Spinal Pain

Remember that the pelvis is large, moves as a unit and is relatively immovable compared to the vertebrae above it (Chapter 3). The junction of the pelvis and the lumbar spine, L5/S1, absorbs most of the stress this architecture creates. The tissues at that junction—vertebra, disc, ligaments, fascia, nerves, muscles—respond to this repeated strain by breaking down in various ways such as forming disc bulges or herniations, fascial rigidity or boney changes such as arthritis or ligament tears.

The muscles on either side of the spine (**paraspinal muscles**) are about three to five inches thick and overlap each other, leap-frogging up and down the spine. Remember that most chronic back pain has an Extension Problem—too much arching of the spine—as one of the primary pain patterns. The paraspinal muscles help maintain the arched spine and these muscles increase their tone or tension in response to being chronically activated because of these movement patterns. Sometimes this is **bilateral** (occurring on both sides of the spine) and sometimes this is **unilateral** (occurring on one side of the spine, which usually also indicates a Sidebending Problem). Additionally, the thoracolumbar fascia (a blanket of fascia found in the lower back and pelvis region) contains a high percentage of myofibroblasts and up to 40% SNS nerve endings. In addition to mechanical stressors, this region is therefore likely responsive to emotional or psychological stressors as well.

All of this is due to historic problems that slowly wound through our bodies as compensations developed. This is one of the reasons why solving back or sciatic pain can be perplexing—the original injury triggering this cascade of events may have happened decades ago even if the precipitating event, such as bending over to pick a sock up off the floor, was recent. Logically though, it's highly unlikely that picking up that sock caused whatever structural changes you've seen on your X-rays or MRI (disc bulge, disc herniation, facet joint arthropathy, degenerated disc, etc.). Instead, those changes have been accumulating for a long time, under the radar waiting to be triggered (think back to Chapter 2 where many structural problems are found to be asymptomatic as we age).

By the time you develop chronic back or sciatic pain, several changes have occurred at different functional levels of your body. While this makes intuitive sense (we even have a children's song where "...the foot bone is connected to the...leg bone"...), there is no documentation or research explaining these connections and consequences of biomechanical faults collectively. Medical research and treatment approaches are typically concerned with *isolating* tissues rather than *combining* them using a systems approach. Therefore, system information relating to *how* the body is linked functionally is difficult or impossible to find in research and, consequently, on the internet. Without research to corroborate these functional links (however impossible that task might be given the opposing nature of medical research and system understanding), most medical professionals will dismiss this type of information. However, the high prevalence of chronic musculoskeletal pain in the world is evidence that something has been missing in our approach to solving pain.

These functional maladaptations can be thought of as biomechanical dysfunctions or strain which can lead to decreased oxygen, increased acidity and an increased concentration of molecules that promote inflammation. To put it simply these conditions can create painful **trigger points**—points that refer to pain elsewhere in the body. Incidentally, these

same conditions that create trigger points also increase myofibroblast activity and activation.[42]

Often when pressed, these trigger points will reproduce pain at the site of the complaint of pain further away. For instance, a trigger point found in the outer muscles of the hip might refer to pain in the low back, sciatica extending down the leg, SI joint or any number of other potential areas of pain. Therefore, understanding the functional links that create these trigger points and pain is critical to the short- and long-term resolution of chronic pain.

An example of functional linking is if the left calf muscle is tighter than the right calf which creates excessive left foot flattening (Chapter 12). Over time this stresses the left plantar fascia causing you to unload that left foot to avoid pain. This could potentially cause a Left Sidebending Problem (Chapters 4 and 7) on that side resulting in decreased left gluteal activation (Chapter 11) and/or an elevated left pelvis and depressed left rib cage (hallmarks of a Left Sidebending Problem—Chapter 7). Consequently, this can potentially compress spinal structures on the left side creating sciatic pain that then eventually migrates back down the left leg to the foot. This may take months or years to wind through the body. As the sciatic pain emerges, you would have an MRI scan that shows a disc bulge or facet joint arthritis in the spine as the cause. However, these structural changes can be thought of as *symptoms of functional linking problems* that then contribute to further degradation in the system.

Continuing further up the kinetic chain, because the left rib cage is depressed, the left shoulder blade, which essentially rests on the rib cage, then also becomes depressed. The muscular connections from the shoulder blade to the neck and head (Chapter 14), namely the levator scapula and trapezius muscles, then act on the cervical spine or skull, potentially creating left-sided neck pain, shoulder pain, radicular symptoms down the left arm and/or left-sided headaches. Again, by the time neurological symptoms like radiculopathy occur, structural changes in the spine have developed as a result of these linked systemic problems.

Just as easily, the left plantar fasciitis could have caused left SI joint pain, left low back pain, left hip or knee pain or even an overuse issue on the right side of the body, due to unloading the painful left foot, ultimately breaking down that side instead. This is why it is important to test the body properly, by reviewing elements of the body system, rather than simply basing treatment on the site of pain or what has shown up on an X-ray or MRI.

Reducing tension and improving movement out of these reflexive/fascial/movement pain patterns while addressing the source problems, disperses forces among additional tissues and joints. This naturally improves range of motion and strength in the areas that have become too tight or weak—in other words, it introduces suppleness. Clinically this rapidly reduces chronic pain as vulnerable tissues are no longer absorbing excessive biomechanical stresses. Remember that pain is simply an indication that something is wrong at that moment. If that problem is fixed, then chronic pain associated with that problem will immediately reduce, in my experience.

Section 2 offers tests for the source of various problems that functionally link to other areas of the body. In other words, these tests will expose hidden sources of tension, weakness or tightness that lock the body into the pain patterns described in Chapters 2, 3 and 4.

Your Pain Pattern Lesson

Pain is a message from your body that something is wrong. Your body is constantly adapting, for the better or worse, in response to problems and in finding solutions. You now understand that different parts of the body are functionally linked to other parts. The following chapters in Section 2 will test various functional links and provide a framework to understand and solve your specific pain pattern.

Section 2   **Practical Applications and Testing**

Section 1 introduced the fundamentals of how our bodies are put together and negotiate our environment. Think of this as the vocabulary and grammar your body uses to communicate. Patterns of movement, fascia and/or reflexes integrate into our postural control using muscle tone or tension to successfully complete tasks efficiently and automatically. Essentially this is how your vocabulary and grammar are internalized and expressed in the world.

This section offers testing to more precisely unravel the subconscious negotiations your brain and body have been making until now. Here you will gain a practical understanding of larger hidden forces feeding the three pain patterns introduced in Section 1: Extension, Flexion, and Sidebending. Consider this as the practical laboratory portion of your course.

You'll notice that most of the tests in this section are unilateral, meaning you will test one side of your body and then the other. Especially if your chronic pain is on one side, there are likely hidden asymmetries in how you use your body at the root of your pain which have led to imbalances in strength and length of muscles, as well as structural changes. When performing the tests in this section, focus on the *quality* of how each side of your body performs the test, rather than simply *your ability* to perform the test successfully. Remember, your brain is wired for short-term success and will subconsciously adjust your technique to assure completion of the test. *These subtle negotiations are likely hiding the sources of your pain.* Move slowly and thoughtfully by removing distractions and focusing on *how* you perform the tests.

To this end, you will learn a lot about your body if you perform the tests in front of a mirror or, even better, video yourself. This allows you to become a more objective observer of your function. Interestingly, when I meet with people who have performed these tests and not found anything wrong with their bodies, I typically find many errors that they simply haven't noticed. I help them see these errors by slowing them down and making them focus on *how their bodies are actually conducting the tests.* Inevitably, once I help them with this, they are amazed they didn't see the errors themselves.

As long as you can become aware of *how* you are, you can change *who* you are. Transformation can then happen at any moment once you understand what needs to be changed.

I would like to mention that no test or exercise should cause pain. If it does, this is yet another way your body is trying to communicate where a problem resides. Rather than simply giving up, be creative and try modifying the test or exercise first by making it easier in some way. For instance, with the Single Leg Standing Test featured in Chapter 8, if you can't stand up with one leg, then use a hiking pole in one hand to help you keep your balance. If you do this, pay attention to how much you rely on that hiking pole for each side of the test. Do you have to make the same accommodations for both sides of your body?

Also, if the test is causing pain, take a moment to review the information in this book to understand *why* that test might cause pain. First of all, have you performed it precisely? Second, is your body compensating for a deficiency which is then causing the pain? If you are performing the test perfectly and there are no compensations, the test is then exposing a tightness or weakness at the root of your pain.

Please record your answers in the results section of each test—regardless of whether they make sense to you. There are several tests in this section and if you don't actually record your answers, you'll likely forget your results. This will help you review your results and understand the elements feeding your chronic pain.

One of the biggest errors that will most likely hold you back from discovering sources of pain is that you will base your judgements about these tests on what past practitioners have told you or what you've uncovered on the internet. If that information was accurate with regards to your pain, you wouldn't be reading this book because your pain would already be resolved. So take a deep breath and clear your mind of what you think you know about your pain. Instead discover what actually is the case regarding your pain problems by recording your results objectively.

Please perform the tests and record your answers BEFORE reading the results of what the tests mean. This is because many people alter their responses to reflect what they believe the results should be, based on their understanding of their pain. Again, you are interested in the *truth* of what your body is telling you rather than your *belief* of what is so. Therefore, approach the tests objectively, recording your responses, before reading the interpretations of what the test results mean.

Finally, in many of the chapters in Section 2, you will see a 🎥 symbol after a title or description. This means you can watch a video of that test or exercise at www.rickolderman.com, and then select the "Books" tab to find the *Pain Patterns* book. Once there, enter the code PainPatterns to unlock the material.

Chapter 6 Testing for Extension or Flexion Problems

Client Connection

Ann suffered from back pain that had confounded health providers for 35 years. Our initial examination revealed that she had an Extension Problem at the root of her pain. We then identified the reasons for this pattern. Primary among them was her habit of locking her knees when standing or walking (Chapter 11), in conjunction with tight thigh muscles (Chapter 9). Within two weeks, Ann's back pain had been reduced by 80% and eventually 100%, after we addressed the other contributors to her Extension Problem pattern.

Extension/Flexion Problem Test

Lie down on the floor on your back with your legs straight (Figure 6.1a). If you are unable to get on the floor, then lie down on your bed or couch. A firmer surface is better, as it gives you more feedback about your pattern of problems. Feel free to put a pillow under your head for comfort. Stay in this position for 30 seconds. Note any low back discomfort.

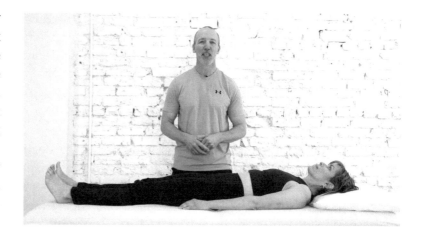

Figure 6.1a Extension or Flexion Test. Knees straight. 🎥

After 30 seconds, bend both knees while keeping the feet flat on the floor and hold that position for another 30 seconds (Figure 6.1b). Your back should feel different in this position when compared to the first position, with your legs straight. If you feel no difference in the level of discomfort in your back, bring both knees to your chest (one at a time) and hug them there with your arms for another 30 seconds (Figure 6.1c). Then you may lower your legs one at a time.

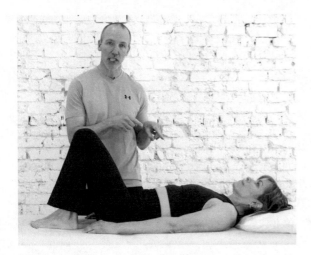

| **Figure 6.1b** Knees bent position.

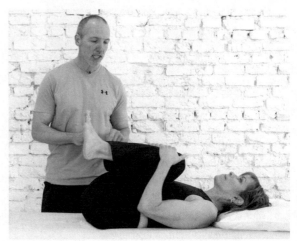

| **Figure 6.1c** Knees to chest position.

| **Your Results** | *Select your answer below* |

✎. __ *My back/sciatica pain felt better with my legs straight.*

✎. __ *My back/sciatica pain felt better with my legs bent.*

Interpreting Your Results

Which position feels better for your back: legs straight or knees bent? In my clinical experience, 99% of people will respond that their back feels better with knees bent. This means you have an Extension Problem—one where your back is too arched, or you have too many forces trying to pull your back into an arch. As changing the position of your legs affects these forces, then it is likely there are issues occurring in your legs and pelvis that are affecting your spine.

The degree of your Extension Problem can be determined by how much you need to bend your knees to make your back feel better. Less bending means you have milder forces acting on your spine, whereas if you must bring your knees to your chest to feel better, then you have more significant issues pulling your spine into extension that need to be addressed.

If your back felt better with your legs straight and felt more painful with your knees bent then you likely have a Flexion Problem. However, these problems are very rare in chronic back pain cases—I see perhaps one case a year in my clinic.

False Response

I have discovered that many of you think or assume your back *should* feel better with your legs straight, and so you give a false response. This is why it is important to take the 60 seconds to feel the truth of what your body is telling you, rather than assume what is true. Your assumptions, likely influenced by past practitioners and online searches, can create barriers to healing. So, start with a clean slate and figure this out beginning with this simple test. If you believe you have a Flexion Problem, please perform the test once more to confirm this. Remember, you are testing whether your back feels *less pain* with your legs straight or your knees bent when lying down.

What Your Test Results Mean

Regardless of what has shown up on your X-rays and MRIs or what you have been told is the source of your back, sciatic or SI joint pain, if bending your knees during this test made your symptoms feel better, then your biomechanics are strongly affecting or perpetuating your pain. This is because in the 60 seconds it took to perform this simple test, you have not changed any of those structural findings in your scans— that would be impossible. Instead, you have changed the forces acting on your spine and, by extension, those structures. I typically lay it out to my patients like this: the things that are causing your pain are likely also causing those structural findings on your scans, which are now also contributing to your pain. This is a critical concept to absorb from this book.

How to Fix an Extension Problem

Unlocking Your Knees 🎥

There are many causes of Extension Problems, however the most consistent is that those of you with this problem tend to lock your knees straight when standing or walking (Figure 6. 2). Test this idea out by standing for three minutes. Most of you will begin locking one or both knees backward after about a minute, if not sooner. This conserves energy by allowing us to bear weight through our joints rather than using our leg muscles to hold us up.

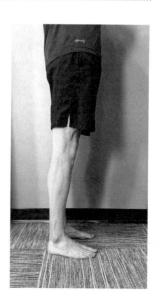

Figure 6.2
Locking knees straight
contributes to Extension Problems.

Notice that when your knees are locked backward, your lower back arches more and likely you'll feel more tension in the lower back muscles. Simply unlocking your knees just a little removes the arch and the low back tension (Figure 6.3).

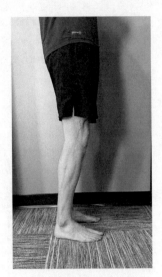

Figure 6.3 Unlocking knees when standing and walking reduces Extension Problem patterns.

Because this is a subconscious habit, I have found that placing a piece of tape on the backs of the knees serves as a prompt, alerting you to the fact you have just locked your knees (Note: Knee Taping is also found in Chapter 11). This has been very effective at changing this pain-causing habit (Figure 6.4). Typically, pain associated with this habit will reduce within 24 hours and the habit itself will be changed in 3–5 days if you are focused on changing this behavior.

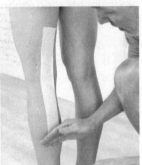

Figure 6.4 Taping the backs of the knees can help cue you to unlock your knees more frequently.

How to Fix a Flexion Problem

Lifting the Rib Cage 🎥
Flexion Problems are quite rare, however understanding that this means that your lower spine is too flat will help you fix it. Central to this pattern is a poor posture strategy resulting in deconditioned lumbar paraspinal muscles (muscles lining both sides of the low back). Therefore, you must slightly increase the arch of your low back or increase the muscle tone of the paraspinal muscles of the low back. Those of you with a Swayback Posture (Chapter 2) will also benefit from this exercise.

Stand up and place one hand on your chest and the other on your belly (Figure 6.5). Inhale gently and feel your rib cage rise. Exhale and feel your rib cage lower again. Now inhale gently again, feeling your rib cage rise. This time, when exhaling, allow it to lower again *but not all the way*—hold your rib cage up higher by perhaps a millimeter or a centimeter. However, feel free to exhale completely.

Notice that your stomach muscles have slightly engaged now. They may feel a little firmer than usual under the hand on your belly. This

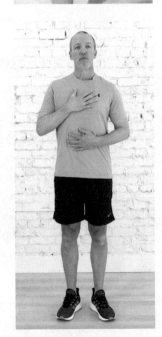

Figure 6.5 Lifting the rib cage.

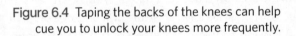

is your core holding up your rib cage. The core muscles will activate just enough to achieve this more ideal posture—you need not consciously contract the core muscles. Instead, simply hold your rib cage up slightly higher than normal. You will feel your low back muscles gently engage to help you with this. You may need to experiment with just how much will reduce your back pain due to a Flexion Problem.

Lastly, relax your arms by your sides. Do not use your shoulders to help arch your back, as this is an artificial means of achieving posture. Basically, the more you use your shoulders, the less you will use your core muscles. Using the shoulders to achieve posture can contribute to chronic neck pain or headaches (see Chapter 14). Therefore, this exercise can also be useful for those types of pain.

Client Connection

Andy had suffered back pain on and off for the past seven years. Lately it was more on than off. We discovered he had a Flexion Problem primarily caused by his poor posture and bending strategy. Once he implemented the Lifting the Rib Cage recommendation, his back pain significantly reduced within the week. This initially required frequent reminders, so I asked him to wear his watch on the opposite wrist, which became a constant reminder to check in on his posture and correct it. After about three weeks, he was able to move his watch back to the original wrist as he had developed better posture that solved his pain.

Clinical Pearl

While counterintuitive, it is possible to have both an Extension and Flexion Problem at the same time. From a chronic back pain perspective, most of you will have an Extension Problem as the primary pain pattern driving your pain. However, on occasion a temporary acute disc problem can arise due to accidents or poor body mechanics. As mentioned in Chapter 2, Flexion Problems tend to relate to disc bulges or herniations. Therefore, solving acute disc episodes will likely involve temporarily treating them as Flexion Problems until they resolve. Once the acute episode has calmed down, you will be left with an Extension Problem pattern feeding chronic back or sciatic pain. ➡

➡ During these acute disc episodes, lying on your stomach (prone position) and often with a pillow under the chest to bring the spine into an extended position, will help reduce disc-related acute spinal pain (see Figure 6.6). This position will normally irritate spinal pain due to Extension Problems. However, as the acute pain resolves, the degree of spinal extension to reduce pain will become less and less—usually over the course of a few days or a week. Once the acute disc episode is resolved completely, you will then be able to continue to address your chronic back or sciatic pain by treating it as an Extension Problem.

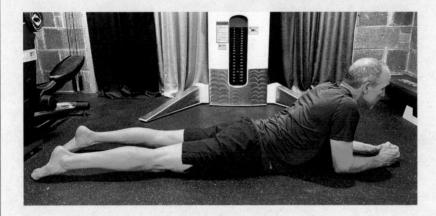

Figure 6.6 Prone position to reduce disc-related Flexion Problems.

Your Pain Pattern Lesson

Almost all back, sciatic or SI joint pain has, at its root, a fundamental problem of too much or too little arching of the spine. Often the sources of these problems are found in the lower body, for instance when locking the knees. Solving the reasons for this pattern will be a step in the right direction to solve your pain.

Chapter 7   Testing for Sidebending Problems

Client Connection

Angie had chronic right-sided back pain and SI joint pain. She had been told by her medical team that she had scoliosis, a disc bulge, a leg-length discrepancy and facet joint arthropathy ("facet joints" are where your vertebrae interact with each other, while "arthropathy" refers to disease of a joint) on the right side of her spine and was recommended cortisone shots to relieve her pain once or twice a year, as necessary. She was also told that her right **quadratus lumborum** (QL) was tight or spasmed. The QL attaches from the ilium of the pelvis to the lumbar vertebrae and lowest rib. It is often blamed for one-sided back pain or sciatica.

We discovered that she had a Right Sidebending Problem and fixed her gait pattern in a large part by implementing the *Reaching While Walking* exercise below, together with the gluteal recommendations found in Chapter 11. We also addressed a previously unknown problem in her right foot and ankle (Chapter 12). In three weeks, she had corrected the right-sided weakness and tightness that caused the collapse of her right side during gait and her pain was 95% eliminated.

Sidebending Problems relate to the Withdrawal/Crossed Extensor Reflex pattern discussed in Chapter 4. They involve one side of a pelvis being higher than the other and one side of the rib cage being lower than the other. These problems relate to one-sided back pain, sciatica, and SI joint pain. They occur because of asymmetries in tightness, strength, or usage patterns typically found in the lower body. There are two ways to test for this problem.

Sidebending Problem Tests

The Picture Test

Remove your shirt and stand naturally. Take a picture of your back from the bottom of your buttocks to the tops of your shoulders (Figures 7.1a and 7.1b). Study your image to see if you have a larger crease on one side of your waist than the other, similar to those seen in Figures 7.1a and 7.1b. Look more closely and you might notice that your pelvis is higher on the same side of the larger crease. The Sidebending Problem is named for the side with the crease (or elevated pelvis). In the figures, both patients have Left Sidebending Problems. The side of the crease is typically the side that is experiencing one-sided back pain, sciatic pain, or SI joint pain.

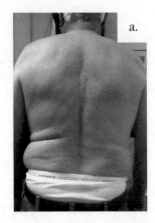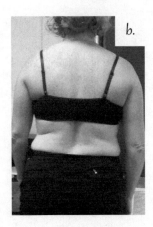

Figure 7.1 These images show Left Sidebending Problems indicated by a larger crease on the left side. Close inspection shows an elevated pelvis on the left side in both cases. Typically, the rib cage is lower on the creased side as well.

Your Results	Select your answer below
	✎ __ My pain is on the left/right side (circle one).
	✎ __ My pain is central.
	In your image, which side has a larger waist crease or which side of the pelvis seems to be higher? Mark one.
	✎ __ My left-side waist has a larger crease than my right and/or the left side of my pelvis seems to be higher than the right side.
	✎ __ My right-side waist has a larger crease than my left and/or the right side of my pelvis seems to be higher than the left side.
	✎ __ I have no crease and my pelvis is level.
	Does your pain correspond to the side with the Sidebending Problem?
	✎ __ Yes
	✎ __ No

If **Yes**, you now understand the pattern/reasoning behind your pain.

If **No**, then you may want to use the Hands-On technique below to confirm your Sidebending Problem pattern or read the Complex Sidebending Pattern information below.

The Hands-On Test 🎥

This test requires more skill and someone to help you. Physical therapists, chiropractors, massage therapists or MDs would be the best people to help you test for this pattern. However, many health or fitness professionals are comfortable and skilled with assessing landmarks on the body including personal trainers, yoga or Pilates instructors. Please give these instructions to them so they understand the proper technique to assess pelvic and rib cage height.

Ask your helper to kneel behind you and place their hands on the tops of the most lateral (side) portion of your pelvis, which are also called the **iliac crests** (the iliac crests are where your hands would be if you were resting with hands on hips). Their eyes should roughly be level with the tops of your pelvis, and they should press their hands into your fleshy waist, towards your spine to get an accurate reading. Compare the height of the iliac crests with the left- and right-hand side and note which one is higher (Figure 7.2).

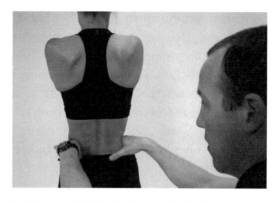

Figure 7.2 Hands-On method of determining a Sidebending Problem.

Your helper can now simply slide their fingers up towards the head, still pressing towards the spine through the waist and feel the lowest rib of your ribcage. Usually, the lowest rib is only about an inch or less from the top of the iliac crest. Note which side is lower. Typically, it is the same side as the higher pelvis for the reasons described previously.

Your Results	Select your answer below
	✎. __ My left pelvis is higher and my left ribs are lower, so I have a Left Sidebending Problem.
	✎. __ My right pelvis is higher and my right ribs are lower, so I have a Right Sidebending Problem.
	✎. __ The left/right (circle one) side of my pelvis is higher and the ribs on the opposite side ribs are lower, so I have a Complex Sidebending Problem. This is indicative of congenital scoliosis, which can also be helped with this information.

Interpreting Your Results

This pelvic asymmetry is often blamed on a difference in the length of the legs, aka leg-length discrepancy. In fact, many practitioners will measure this difference in pelvic height when patients are standing, to confirm the leg-length discrepancy. However, this could not be further from the truth in most cases. In my 25+ years as a physical therapist, I may have seen fewer than five people with actual leg-length discrepancies. However, I have probably been told by hundreds of patients when they enter my clinic that they have a leg-length discrepancy which was measured by a healthcare professional. In my book, *Solving the Pain Puzzle* (McFarland, 2023), I even tell the story of a woman who had full-length lower body X-rays to prove her claim to me, which was quickly refuted with a correct measurement and Sidebending Problem correction.

Many of these people have been sold expensive shoe lifts or foot orthotics to correct for this apparent discrepancy. This is an artificial correction that usually fails to solve pain over time because the conditions creating the Sidebending Problem have not been addressed or corrected.

Clinical Pearl

The medical term for a spine experiencing a lateral curve is "scoliosis." This does not distinguish between **functional scoliosis**, meaning one caused by how you use your body and which is easily corrected, or **congenital scoliosis**—scoliosis you are born with. Functional scoliosis usually involves just one lateral curve—often referred to as a C-curve. Congenital scoliosis usually involves two curves in opposite directions and is referred to as an S-curve. Both are treatable.

Because an MRI or X-ray report does not often distinguish between the two types, medical providers are left to simply report that the patient has scoliosis, without further explanation. Because most patients don't understand the different types of scoliosis, they then assume they have congenital scoliosis with an S-curve. Both types of scoliosis can be considered Sidebending Problems.

Congenital scoliosis (which I refer to as a **Complex Sidebending Problem**), is often correctible to a large degree and involves a higher pelvis on one side and a lower rib cage on the other. There is a special approach to solving congenital scoliosis called the Schroth Method. I recommend seeking out a practitioner if you have this type of scoliosis and wish to try to correct it. The information in this book and my home programs can help you with this, too.

I have found that both types of scoliosis are magnified by poor movement habits. Correcting these movement habits reverses functional scoliosis and, to a degree, slows down or reverses the progression of congenital scoliosis.

How to Fix a Sidebending Problem

Reaching While Walking 🎥

The results of this correction are most dramatic if you have measured your Sidebending Problem using the hands-on method first. This is because skin and other soft tissues often have adapted to this pattern and will not change immediately, even if the pelvis and rib cage have been corrected. Results are best seen measuring with the hands before and after this simple exercise to confirm the correction.

First, determine the side of your Sidebending Problem. For the sake of demonstration, let's assume it is on the right side, opposite Figures 7.1a and 7.1b, above.

Simply raise your right arm up in the air, as if reaching for the ceiling, and walk 20 steps. Each time you bear weight through your right leg, emphasize lengthening your right waist by reaching up to the ceiling a little more (Figure 7.3). Walk slowly. If you cannot reach your right hand up to the ceiling because of, say, a shoulder problem, simply putting the hand on top of your head also does the trick.

Now have your assistant re-measure the Right Sidebending Problem—the pelvis and rib cage should now be level or significantly improved.

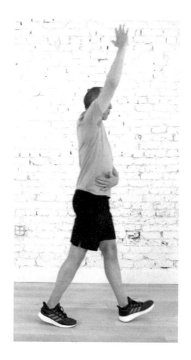

Figure 7.3 Reaching while walking to correct a Right Sidebending Problem.

Your Results	*Select your answer below*
	🖊 __ *My pelvis and ribs are level after performing the Reaching While Walking correction. I do not currently have a Sidebending Problem.*
	🖊 __ *My pelvis and ribs are more level after performing the Reaching While Walking correction but not completely level. I still have a slight Sidebending Problem. In this case, repeat the Reaching While Walking correction to see if your pelvis and rib cage level completely.*
	🖊 __ *My pelvis and ribs are the same as before performing the Reaching While Walking correction. I have the same degree of Sidebending Problem. In this case, try it one more time and re-measure. This has never failed to correct a Sidebending Problem in almost 15 years of using this method clinically. While this exercise is much more successful correcting functional scoliosis, it also helps correct Sidebending Problems associated with congenital scoliosis.*

What has this taught you? That your Side-bending Problem has a lot to do with how you are walking—otherwise walking would never fix a scoliotic curve, even temporarily. Simply performing this maneuver for ten or 20 steps every time you get up from a chair for the next two or three days should significantly reduce or eliminate your one-sided pain associated with a Sidebending Problem. However, there may be other problems feeding that pain pattern which will also need to be corrected from a long-term perspective.

> **Clinical Pearl**
>
> Sidebending Problems are often classified as Rotation Problems in medicine because a lateral spinal curve causes spinal rotation to the opposite direction (see Chapter 4). As a physical therapist, I was taught to correct the rotated vertebrae. Clinically, I was never successful at this, as the problem would always return. Once I discovered the Sidebending Problem pattern and realized that this was the driver of vertebral rotation, I began fixing that instead. Doing so, what I had considered to be rotation-related spinal pain melted away.

I have found that 80-90% of Sidebending Problems in my clinic occur due to old, forgotten injuries to the leg on the *same side* of the Sidebending Problem. In 10-20% of the cases, the Sidebending Problem is in response to a lower body problem in the *opposite leg*. You will determine which side of your body is likely creating your Sidebending Problem in Chapter 8.

Your Pain Pattern Lesson

Almost all one-sided back pain, sciatica, or SI joint pain is associated with asymmetry of the pelvis and rib cage—a Sidebending Problem. To permanently solve a Sidebending Problem, you will need to address the asymmetrical lower body problems feeding it. Begin paying attention to standing/walking/turning activities that seem to promote this pattern. Sitting behaviors also feed this pattern. The remaining tests in this book will also help you home in on these problems.

Chapter 8 Testing for Lower Body Compensations

Client Connection

Cathy was an elite marathon runner who had wrestled with right-sided back pain for years and was told she had a right-sided disc bulge, arthritic changes in her spine, and degenerative disc disease. Her training focused on her right trunk and leg strength. We discovered that she had a Right Sidebending Problem (Chapter 7). However, this was due to a compensation pattern from her left leg, which was 50% weaker than her right, unbeknownst to her or her medical team or trainers. She was then able to trace her original left leg injury to a high school incident decades ago. Once she corrected her left leg injury and weakness, her right-sided pain reduced by 80% in approximately four weeks while she was still training.

You have learned that most spine, pelvic and especially lower body pain can be traced back to problems in the legs which affect how we walk, bend, exercise, or sit. Regardless of where your pain is, it is critical to understand whether an historical leg problem is on the same side of the body where you feel your pain or if you are compensating for a problem on the other side of your body. I have devised two very simple tests to help narrow down where to look for these issues. Please perform the Single Leg Standing and Side Plank Tests below but ✋ ***DO NOT read the "Interpreting Your Results" section without doing those two tests first as this will likely have an influence on your results***.

Your Results	*Select your answer below*
✎ __ My pain is on my right/left side (circle one).
✎ __ My pain is central.

Single Leg Standing Test 🎥

Find a chair that you believe you can stand up from using just one leg. Some people will use a kitchen chair, but others might need a higher chair, like a bar stool. Feel free to put pillows or books on the seat of the chair to alter the height in order to perform the test. You will *only need to perform one repetition on each leg but that one repetition should be challenging*—this way your results will be clearer. So, adjust the height of the chair appropriately. Testing multiple chairs and heights will affect this test. Therefore, try to determine the correct height without testing it first—take your best guess.

If your balance is an issue, feel free to use a broom or walking stick for stability or place your chair in a doorway so you can use your hands for balance. The only rule about this is *you must use the same hand to help steady yourself as the leg you are standing up with*. For instance, if you are standing up using the *left* leg, you must use the *left* hand to help steady you on your left side. If you are standing up with the right leg, you will then need to switch the stick to the right hand to help steady yourself. Use as little help as possible with your hands to steady yourself—this will give a more accurate result. Lastly, if you are using your hands to help, *pay attention to how much each hand is helping*. I strongly recommend you video record your test on your phone to analyze your results—the camera should be facing you from the front.

Here's the test: sit on the chair and scoot to the front to make it easier to stand up. Stand up, then sit down using just one leg (it does not matter which leg you choose). The other foot should not touch the floor during this test (Figures 8.1a and 8.1b). Only do one repetition. Once you have done one repetition with one leg, do one repetition with the other leg. Note how easy or difficult this was for each leg.

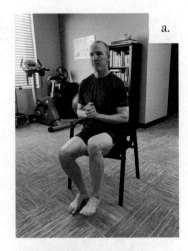

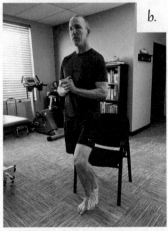

Figures 8.1 Single leg standing test.

Your Results	*Select your answer below*
	✎ __ I stood up using my Right leg first.
	✎ __ I stood up using my Left leg first.
	✎ __ My Right/Left (circle one) leg felt stronger than my other leg. For the purposes of this test, consider that leg to be 100% strong.

Compared to my strong leg (in the choice above which is 100%), **my weak leg felt ___ % as strong as my strong leg**.

Side Plank Test 🎥

This is a more aggressive test. You will only perform one repetition. Feel free to skip this test, if you feel it is too difficult or will cause significant pain. You may be able to get enough information from the other tests in this book to understand the sources feeding your pain pattern and tension.

Lie down on your left or right side on the floor (while the floor is preferable, use your bed if the floor is too difficult to manage—a firmer surface is more ideal). Prop yourself up on your elbow, making sure it is underneath your shoulder. Your other arm and hand will be resting on your top hip. Your legs and feet should be stacked on top of each other.

Simply lift your hips into the air to create a Side Plank position where your legs are not touching the floor (Figure 8.2a). Note how much of your bottom leg is touching the floor when you do this (is it just the foot, the foot and ankle, the lower leg too?). If

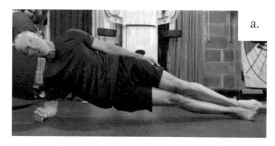

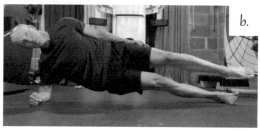

Figure 8.2 Side Plank Test beginning (a) and lifting the top leg (b).

possible, now raise your top leg in the air a few inches, maintaining your side plank position for a few seconds (Figure 8.2b). Note the level of difficulty doing this. Lower your leg and hips back down.

Repeat with the other leg.

Your Results	*Select your answer below*
	✎ ___ *I performed the Side Plank Test (position a) lying on my Right/Left (circle one) side first.*
	✎ ___ *Sideplanking while on my right/left (circle one) side was easier. We will call this 100% strong.*
	✎ ___ *Sideplanking on my stronger side, I could/could not (circle one) raise my leg (position b) once in the Side Plank position.*
	✎ ___ *Sideplanking on my weaker side, I could/could not (circle one) raise my leg (position b) once in the Side Plank position.*
	✎ ___ *Sideplanking on my weaker side felt ___% weaker compared to my stronger side.*

Interpreting the Single Leg Standing Test 📹

The logic is quite simple in interpreting your results from this test. Your brain is wired for short-term success and so it will subconsciously choose your stronger leg first to stand up with—*regardless of whether it is painful or not.* Look at your results to confirm which leg you used first.

If your stronger, or first leg, was your pain-free side, then you are probably not compensating for a problem on the other side of your body. This is because it is logical that your non-painful side would also be your stronger side.

If your stronger, or first leg, was also your painful side, then you are likely compensating for some older injury or problem in the other leg that has made that other leg weaker. This is because your subconscious mind knows the non-painful leg is weaker and can't perform as well. Therefore, it will choose the painful leg because it will be more successful. How much are you compensating? Roughly the percentage difference felt between the two legs. So, if your weak leg has only 50% of the strength of your stronger leg, then roughly 50% of your body's load is being transferred to your stronger leg, which is now breaking down under that added load and creating pain due to overuse.

I have found that 80-90% of the time the first leg someone uses is their non-painful, stronger side. In 10-20% of the cases, there is a compensation pattern happening whereby the painful leg is actually the stronger leg (the first leg you use to stand up with) which has been carrying too much load and is likely breaking down.

Your Results	*Select your answer below*
✎. ___ My painful side is my stronger side, therefore the problems feeding my pain are likely originating on the opposite side of my body.	
✎. ___ My painful side is my weaker side, therefore the problems feeding my pain are likely happening on that same, painful side.	

Solving Single Leg Standing Strength Asymmetry

Sitting and Standing

An easy way to begin correcting this asymmetry can be achieved when standing up and sitting down in a chair. If you are sitting, simply position your strong foot forward a few inches so the weaker foot is closer to the chair. Now when you stand up, you will be forced to use the weaker leg more than the stronger leg which will naturally strengthen the weaker leg throughout the day (Figure 8.3). The same will be true if you use this staggered stance before sitting down, to recruit the weaker leg more.

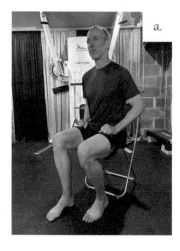
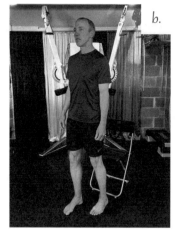
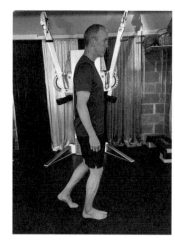

Figure 8.3 Stagger your feet when standing from sitting (a) and sitting from standing (b). The foot closest to the chair will bear more weight.

Figure 8.4 Stagger your stance and bear more weight on the forward leg with a slightly bent knee to naturally strengthen your leg while performing common activities.

Standing

When standing in line at a bank, preparing food in the kitchen, brushing your teeth or cleaning dishes, stagger your weaker leg forward a few inches and weight-shift onto that leg, keeping the knee slightly bent (Figure 8.4). This will load that weaker leg more, strengthening it throughout the day. Be sure you are standing tall and lengthened through the waist when using that weaker leg to avoid perpetuating a sidebending pattern.

Interpreting the Side Plank Test 📹

The Side Plank Test challenges your lateral (side) body strength including your ankle, hip, knee, pelvic and waist muscles. Because a Sidebending Problem involves a lateral curve, this test helps you see if the curve formation is, in part, due to weakness in your lateral musculature. Very similar to the Single Leg Standing Test above, it is important to understand if your lateral strength is weaker on the same side of the Sidebending Problem or on the opposite side.

As in the Single Leg Standing Test, subconsciously you will likely begin on your stronger side. For instance, if you began by lying on your right side (Figure 8.2a), then your brain believes your right side is stronger than your left for this test. Lifting your left leg up in the air (Figure 8.2b) after you have assumed the Side Plank posture stresses the right lateral musculature even more. An inability to lift the left leg in this instance does not mean your left leg is weaker. Instead, it means that your right lateral musculature is unable to stabilize your body in order to lift the left leg.

Solving Lateral Strength Asymmetry

Standing Hip Strengthening 🎥

Lateral weakness is especially important during standing and walking. If you need balance help, for instance holding a pole during this exercise, please use the pole in the same hand as the leg you are standing on. Therefore, if you are standing on your right leg, you will have a pole in your right hand for additional balance and vice versa.Performing this exercise in front of a mirror or making a video of yourself from the front will help you see whether you are symmetrical or not.

Level 1

Stand on one leg with the other foot about 1/2" off the floor (Figure 8.5). Your stance knee should be soft. Your hips should not jut out to the side. Your trunk should be tall, and your waist is lengthened, not sidebent. Use a pole in your hand if necessary. Hold for 30 seconds, then switch legs. Repeat twice, 3–5x/day until this is easy, and you are not compensating. In this exercise, you are challenging the stance leg side of your lower body system.

Level 2

Stand as in Level 1. Lift and then move the non-weight-bearing leg out to the side about 6 inches and then back in for 15 repetitions maintaining proper positioning described above (Figure 8.6). Repeat on the other side. Continue repeating for three sets per leg. Perform two- or three-times a day until it becomes easy, and you are not compensating. In this exercise, you are challenging the stance leg side of your lower body system, not the moving leg side.

Level 3

Stand as in level 1 & 2 but this time standing on an exercise tube with both feet and holding the ends of the tube in your hands. Lift and then move the non-weight-bearing leg out to the side about six inches and then back in for 15 repetitions, maintaining proper positioning described above (Figure 8.7). Repeat on the other side. Continue repeating for three sets per leg. Perform two- or three-times per day until it becomes easy, and you are not compensating. In this exercise, you are challenging the stance leg side of your lower body system, not the moving leg side.

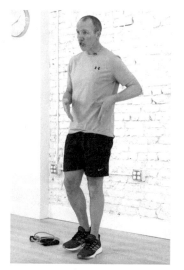 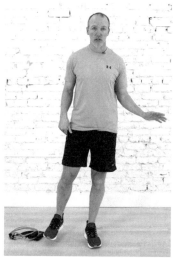 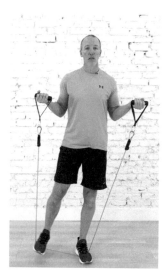

Figure 8.5 Level 1, Standing Hip Strengthening

Figure 8.6 Level 2, Standing Hip Strengthening

Figure 8.7 Level 3, Standing Hip Strengthening

Your Pain Pattern Lesson

Sidebending Problems are typically caused by strength, length, and habit asymmetries in the lower body. This could occur in the form of tighter or weaker muscles on one side and/or be due to older forgotten injuries that no longer cause pain because your brain has created compensations to get around those problems.

Understanding which leg houses older problems that feed your pain will help you rapidly discover exactly where the root problem is. Balancing strength and range of motion between your legs will be important to fix Sidebending Problems. Begin correcting this imbalance by paying attention to and correcting movement habits like standing, bending, and walking to naturally strengthen your weak side. Also pay attention to any asymmetries discovered in the other tests found in this book.

Chapter 9   Testing for Tight Thigh Muscles

Client Connection

Sarah was a gymnast who suffered from chronic low back pain and had a diagnosis of spondylolisthesis—a small fracture in the vertebrae that allows one vertebra to slide forward in relation to the other. Her vertebrae were not stacked on top of each other symmetrically because of the slippage this problem created. Many of her routines required her to kick one or both legs behind her, touching the back of her head with her foot. We discovered that she had an Extension Problem and extremely tight thigh muscles in the front of her legs. This reduced her hip extension (the ability for the thigh bone to move behind the hip) by approximately 40 degrees. Therefore, for her foot to touch the back of her head, she folded her spine backwards into extension, rather than extending her hip behind her. We stretched her front thigh muscles and within two weeks she could perform all routines with no back pain.

Thigh Muscles

One of the muscle groups that can cause significant irritation to the entire lower body system and back are the thigh muscles found on the front of the leg. They are long and powerful and attach to the front of the pelvis. This gives them the potential to deliver significant force directly to the knee, hip, and pelvis. Indirectly, tight or contracted thigh muscles extend their effects to the SI joints and lumbar spine. Tight thigh muscles can tilt the pelvis forward, referred to as **anterior pelvic tilt** (Figure 9.1), or exert continuous force to the pelvis without it tilting forward, which is equally damaging. This can be symmetrical or asymmetrical.

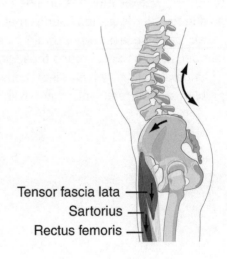

Tensor fascia lata
Sartorius
Rectus femoris

Figure 9.1 Tight thigh muscles contribute to Extension Problems.

Often this muscle group becomes tight either from exercise, response to injuries or pain, or as part of deeper reflex patterns of contraction associated with sitting or standing. If this group becomes tighter on one side than the other, significant rotational torque is then generated through the pelvis, SI joints and lumbar spine contributing to one-sided back pain, sciatica, and SI joint pain (Figure 9.2). This can create Sidebending Problems. Fixing tightness, especially asymmetrical tightness, is often a big key to solving pain associated with these two patterns.

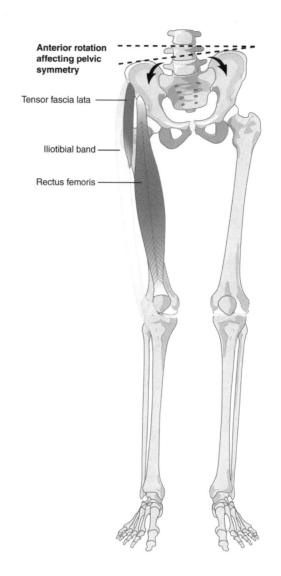

Figure 9.2 Asymmetrical thigh muscle tightness can create rotational torque through the pelvis, SI joint and spine causing Sidebending Problems and other pain.

Thigh Muscle Tightness Test 📹

This test is best done on a firm surface, such as a kitchen countertop, stable dining room table or high coffee table. If none of these are available, then a bed will work. Sit at the edge of the table with a space of about 3-4 inches between the back of the knee and the table edge. Lie back and hug both knees comfortably toward your chest—this position establishes the foundation from which to perform this exercise. If you tested positive for an Extension Problem (Chapter 6), place a pillow under your head. Those with Extension Problems, should find this position very comfortable.

Then move both hands to hold the left knee firmly to your chest—this will protect your back and pelvis during the test. Slowly lower your right leg straight down without allowing it to drift to the outside of your body, in order to keep it in line with your hip joint. Keep the right knee bent to 90 degrees as the leg lowers off the edge of the table (Figure 9.3). Do not force the leg down—just relax and note how far off the table it is and any tightness felt in the front of the right thigh or hip. Hold here for about 10-15 seconds to note tightness and range of motion. If this is painful for your back or pelvis, pull the left knee closer to your chest and/or allow the toes of the right foot to rest on a chair which will support the weight of your leg. If this is painful to your right knee or hip, allow the leg to drift to the outside of your hip. Gradually you can move the leg back to center as these muscles lengthen.

Normal range of motion is for the thigh to naturally rest on the tabletop with the knee bent at 90 degrees and with little to no sense of tightness in the front of the thigh muscles. Note how far your right leg can be lowered down without forcing it.

Bring the right knee back up and hug both knees to your chest to reset your pelvis and lumbar spine before repeating with the left leg. Once completed on both sides, sit up and record your information below.

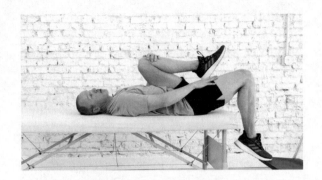

Figure 9.3 Thigh Tightness Test.

Your Results	*Select your answer below*

✎ __ *Both of my legs can be easily lowered down to the tabletop while keeping my knees bent at 90 degrees, while aligned with my hip joint and I do not feel a thigh stretch. This means my thigh muscles are not tight and likely not contributing to my pain.*

✎ __ *My Right/Left/Both (circle one) legs cannot be lowered down to the tabletop while keeping my knee bent at 90 degrees, and while aligned with my hip joint. This means the Right/Left/Both (circle one) side(s) of my thigh muscles are tight. It is also possible that both legs are tight but one is tighter than the other. Note which side is tighter in this case. This may be a significant contributor to your pain, especially if it is one-sided pain.*

How to Fix Tight Thigh Muscles 🎥

To solve this problem, use the same method you did to test for your thigh tightness. Simply hold the stretch to each side for 30–60 seconds and alternate sides twice. Some people will need to support the lowered foot on a chair to unload the weight of the leg from the back and pelvis. Perform this two- or three-times per day until the tightness is corrected and then you can gradually wean yourself off the stretch. Do not force the leg down. When performed correctly, you will likely notice an immediate improvement in your pain level if this is a significant component of your pain pattern. If you have a Sidebending Problem, re-measure that pattern using the Hands-On method to see if it is now corrected.

Your Pain Pattern Lesson

Tight thigh muscles are one of the biggest generators of torque in the lower body and back system and are easily corrected. This muscle group creates Extension Problems by tilting the pelvis forward which consequently causes the low back to arch more. If this is asymmetrical, it can cause a Sidebending Problem or SI joint pain on the side with tighter thigh muscles. Many people will solve their Sidebending Problem when this asymmetry has been corrected. Therefore, pay special attention to correcting asymmetry between the two legs..

Chapter 10   Testing for Twisted Thigh Bones

Client Connection

Carl was an NFL lineman plagued by chronic hip and ankle pain for the previous nine years since beginning college football. His evaluation showed he had one anteverted femur and one retroverted femur. We adjusted his strengthening and pass-blocking form according to these results and his pain evaporated within about one week—while practicing during the season.

Anteversion & Retroversion

The shape of the thigh bones (**femurs**) can cause significant tension in the lower body and back system. There is a spectrum of thigh bone shapes that includes femurs that are twisted inward (**Femoral Anteversion**) and those that are twisted outward (**Femoral Retroversion**— Figures 10.1a and 10.1b). Of course there are thigh bones that are neither. It is very simple to test for this.

Twisty Thigh Bone Test 📹

Lie down on your stomach on the bed or floor. If your back hurts in this position (a sign of an Extension Problem and possibly tight thigh muscles), feel free to put a pillow under your trunk to remove pressure—this reduces arching of the lower spine. Bend both knees so the soles of your feet point toward the ceiling. Now allow both feet to fall to the outside of your body while maintaining your bent knees (Figure 10.2). Note how far your feet can travel outward. Do not force this motion. Remain relaxed. It may be helpful to take a picture of the angles of your legs in this position.

Now straighten your left leg, allowing it to rest on the floor. Keeping the right knee bent, allow the right foot to travel across the center of your body towards the back of your left knee— do not allow your right pelvis to rotate or twist too much with the leg as you do this (Figure 10.3a). Again, do not force this motion, just relax. Note the angle of the right lower leg. Now do the same on the other side: rest your right leg on the floor, bend your left knee and allow it to travel across midline towards the back of the right knee (Figure 10.3b). Note the angle of the left lower leg. It may be helpful to take a picture of the angles of your legs in this position.

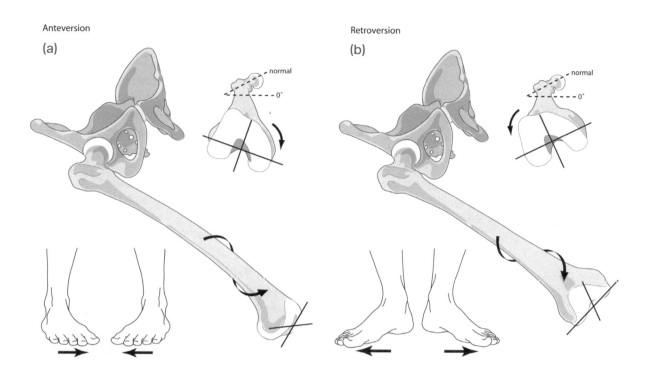

Anteversion
(a)

Retroversion
(b)

Figures 10.1 Femoral anteversion (a) and retroversion (b) are common variances in the shape of thigh bones.

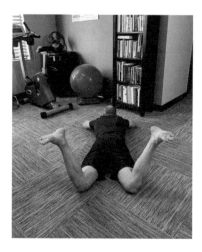

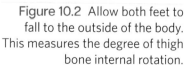

Figure 10.2 Allow both feet to fall to the outside of the body. This measures the degree of thigh bone internal rotation.

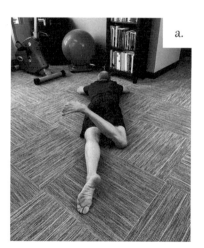

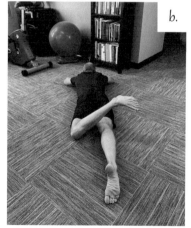

Figure 10.3 Allow one foot to fall to the inside of the body. Then test the other. This measures the degree of thigh bone external rotation.

Results 📹	Select your answer below

✎ __ My legs move outward more than they do inward, which means I likely have Femoral Anteversion (internally rotated thigh bones).

✎ __ My legs move inward, across midline, more than they do outward, which means I likely have Femoral Retroversion (externally rotated thigh bones).

✎ __ My legs move inward and outward roughly the same amount, so I likely have neutral thigh bones and need not consider this as a cause of my pain.

✎ __ My Left/Right (circle one) leg moves more inward (retroversion) and my Left/Right (circle one) moves more outward (anteversion), so my femurs are asymmetrical. If this is the case, pay attention to the femur that is moving *more* in one direction. For instance, if your left thigh bone moves significantly further outward than inward, while the right thigh bone rotates roughly the same amount in both directions, then likely you have an anteverted left thigh bone.

Like all things with the human body, there is a spectrum along which you will reside in this test. If your feet can travel significantly more in one direction than the other, then you have a higher degree of thigh bone rotation in that direction. Men tend to have femoral retroversion (externally rotated thigh bones) and women tend to have femoral anteversion (internally rotated thigh bones). However, this varies to some degree.

How to Fix Pain Associated with Femoral Ante-/Retroversion 📹

It is important to understand that the shape of the thigh bones cannot be changed. Instead, we must change how we use our body, given the knowledge of this phenomenon. The recommendations below have helped my patients eliminate the tension and pain associated with these two conditions.

Retroversion—Turn the Feet Out

Because femoral retroversion involves a thigh bone that is externally rotated, we must then align the foot with the shape of this bone. This removes excessive pain-causing tension in the lower body, pelvic and back system by relaxing the inner thigh muscles (See Deep Front Line of fascia in Chapter 3). To this end, a person with femoral retroversion will need to rotate their feet outward by 3-5 degrees.

The amount of foot rotation can be quickly determined by standing naturally for about 20 seconds, assessing the tension in your legs and back. Next, turn your feet outward 3-5 degrees and note whether your legs and back feel more relaxed. It should be easier to soften your knees. To confirm the effectiveness of this, turn your feet back to their natural standing position (facing forward) and again sense the tension in your legs (especially inner thigh muscles) and back. You will likely now notice the increased tension in your lower body/pelvic/back system that has been subconsciously generated due to past foot positioning. You will also notice that it is more difficult to soften your knees, which leads to other pain pattern problems throughout the lower body and back system (Chapters 6 and 11).

Turning the feet out is pejoratively referred to as "walking like a duck." However, the people who invented this social slur had no knowledge of femoral retroversion. Adopting this movement strategy will involve convincing yourself that this pattern is natural and pain-reducing.

Client Connection

Jim was in his fifties and had intermittent groin pain, especially when he increased his outdoor activities. His evaluation showed he had retroverted femurs, however he stood with his feet facing directly forward. My recommendation to him to stand and walk with feet turned out was met with reluctance. "I don't want to walk like a duck!" he said after our third appointment, but he also reported an 85% improvement in his pain. I consoled him by explaining the angle he was now choosing to use may not be the permanent angle he decided upon. Instead, it's just the angle that is most suitable to dig him out of his years of excessive tension developed from poor walking habits. Eventually he settled on a less severe angle of foot external rotation and continued his activities pain free.

Anteversion–Butt Pumps

Clinical Pearl

In my clinical experience, femoral anteversion occurs significantly more frequently in females. Female athletes also have up to a three-times higher incidence of ACL tears.[43] I believe this is due, in part, to poorly controlled femoral anteversion creating excessive shear forces across the knee joint. Screening for this common phenomenon and creating a program to strengthen and neurologically recruit the gluteal muscles which are external rotators of the thigh bones, together with more precise pronation (foot flattening) control of the foot and ankle, should reduce the risk of these tears due to uncontrolled femoral rotation.

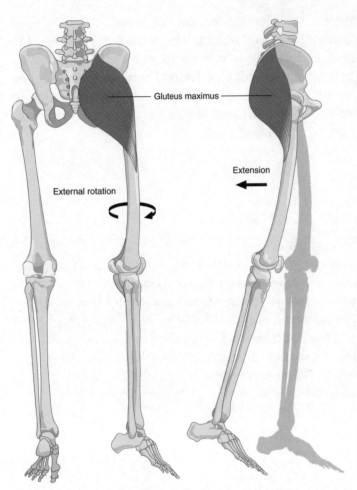

Those with femoral anteversion need to strengthen their **gluteal (butt) muscles** more. The gluteals are external rotators of the legs which then help control excessive internal rotation due to femoral anteversion (Figure 10.4).

Figure 10.4 The gluteus maximus externally rotates the leg and therefore decelerates internal rotation associated with femoral anteversion.

Butt Pumps 📹

Assume a position on your elbows and knees with the spine in a flattened or neutral position. Hold your spine in place by drawing in your belly button. Raise one leg up in the air with the knee bent at 90 degrees by squeezing the glutes on that side. Stop at the point where you feel the maximal contraction of these muscles but without arching the spine (which would contribute to an Extension Problem). Slowly lower the leg about an inch then raise it again (Figure 10.5). Perform this small pump, moving the leg up and down while maintaining the gluteal contraction. Do not lower the leg to the point the gluteals turn off. Make the glutes fatigue. Perform 10–30 repetitions until fatigue, failure or compensations start occurring such as arching the spine or recruiting the hamstrings. Alternate sides for two sets. If this reduces pain or you have a significant deficit, repeat 2–3 times a day.

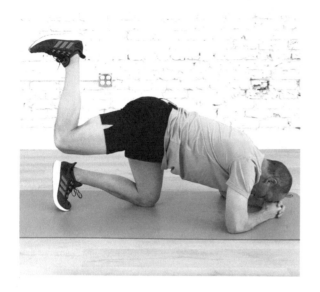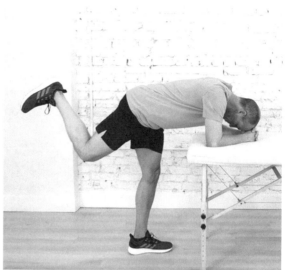

| Figure 10.5 Butt Pumps.

Gluteal Walking

Those with anteverted femurs will need to focus on changing their walking pattern to naturally activate the gluteal muscles better throughout the day (Chapter 11). If you take 10,000 steps a day then you will have activated your gluteal muscles 10,000 repetitions and will have controlled their femoral anteversion consistently throughout the day. Please see Chapter 11 for techniques to achieve this.

Client Connection

Jen suffered from left-sided SI joint pain for over a year. We discovered that both of her legs had anteverted femurs but that her left gluteal muscles were completely turned off during walking (see Chapter 11) while the right gluteal muscles worked better. She also had tight left thigh muscles (see Chapter 9). Stretching her thigh muscles and fixing her walking pattern improved her symptoms by 75%. Butt pumps quickly bumped those results to a 100% reduction in her SI joint pain.

Your Pain Pattern Lesson

Femoral anteversion and retroversion are rarely considered by most providers and may be the missing link you will need to solve your pain. Walking or exercising without understanding the presence of these conditions feeds lower body tension and contributes to Extension or Sidebending Problems. Understanding the shape of your thigh bones is fundamental to reduce chronic lower body and back tension for this reason in many people. It will also improve athletic performance.

Chapter 11   Testing Gluteal Function

Client Connection

Sylvia was in her sixties and suffered from chronic right hip bursitis, a labral tear, and joint pain, especially when gardening and walking along trails. She had been diagnosed with hip arthritis and was scheduled for a hip replacement in two weeks. We discovered that she had anteverted femurs (Chapter 10) and poor gluteal (butt muscle) activation during gait (walking). I recommended butt pumps (Chapter 10) and taught her to improve her gait pattern to naturally turn on her gluteals when walking. Within one week, she was 50% better and canceled her hip replacement surgery. In two more weeks, she was 100% pain-free. Eight months later, she was still pain-free and had returned to enjoying all activities.

The gluteal muscles are some of the strongest in our body and are designed for continuous work. While they fulfill several duties, one of their primary roles is to control the leg and pelvis while walking (Figure 11.1).

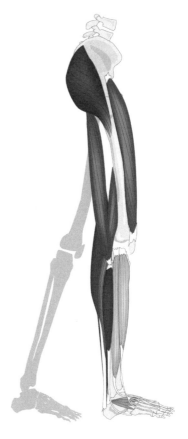

Figure 11.1 Gluteal activation is important during gait to control the thigh bone, hip joint, pelvic orientation, and lumbar spine.

Gluteal Walking Test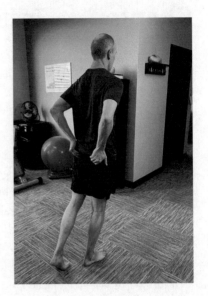

Part 1.
Stand with your fingertips pressing firmly into the center of your butt muscles. Consciously contract your butt muscles by pinching them together. Using your fingertips, feel the firmness of your butt muscles and notice whether both activate at the same time and to the same degree. Consider this a 100% contraction of those muscles.

Part 2.
Relax your butt muscles completely but keep the fingertips firmly pressed into them. Walk naturally for about 20 steps and notice whether you feel your butt muscles naturally turning on while you walk (Figure 11.2).

Figure 11.2 When walking normally, note whether your butt muscles are turning on naturally with each step.

Your Results	*Select your answer below*
	✎. __ *My butt muscles turn on naturally when I walk.*
	✎. __ *I don't feel my butt muscles turn on when I walk.*
	✎. __ *I feel my Right/Left (circle one) butt muscle turn on more than my other one.*

Most people with back, sciatic, SI joint, hip, knee, or foot pain will find their gluteal muscles are not turning on well when they walk. They should activate perhaps 5-10% of the 100% contraction you felt during the first part of this test.

How to Fix Poor Gluteal Function When Walking

Tiptoe Walking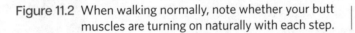
Place your fingertips firmly on your butt muscles again while walking 20 steps on your tiptoes. Notice that your butt muscles are now turning on more than when you first tested them during normal walking—this is how they should be activating naturally when you walk correctly (Figure 11.3). Slowly lower your heels back down to the floor with fingertips remaining on your butt muscles to monitor them. You should notice that the gluteals are working better now,

at least for a few steps. They are turning on because you are walking correctly, not because you are consciously contracting them. There are two primary reasons they are remaining on:

1. Your knees are soft (slightly bent), rather than locked straight when the foot strikes the ground, and
2. Your body is moving forward with the advancing foot, rather than allowing the advancing foot and leg to move forward while your body remains behind.

Every time you stand up from a chair, bed, toilet, or car, take a few steps on your tiptoes to fix your walking pattern and activate your gluteals naturally. After a few days you should notice that the gluteals turn on even without tiptoe walking. Essentially you are changing your gait pattern to fix your lower body system.

Ice-Skate Gluteal Walking 📹

This technique involves pretending that you are ice-skating. Place your fingertips on your butt muscles and slightly bend forward while stepping forward with one leg—just like ice skating. The advancing leg can even move to the outside of the body when pushing off (Figure 11.4). To ice-skate walk correctly, you must commit to the advancing leg whose knee is bent by allowing the body to be over that foot at the moment of foot strike. Feel the butt muscles engage naturally when this happens. If you do not feel these muscles engage then crouch lower and/or bend forward more while "skating" by bending your knees more until they activate—they will feel firmer. Continue for a few steps like this, ice skating around your room and feel the gluteal muscles engage at foot strike.

Once you feel the gluteal muscles activate for a few steps, gradually become taller as you continue skating around your room. At some point, as you become taller, your butt muscles will cease to engage. You will likely not be fully upright when this happens. Continue practicing this technique until you are able to be fully upright and feel that the gluteal muscles are activating naturally at foot strike.

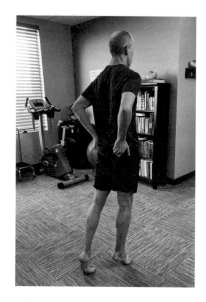

Figure 11.3 Tiptoe walking can help turn on butt muscles naturally.

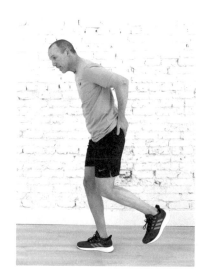

Figure 11.4 Ice-skate walking can help turn on butt muscles naturally.

Why Do Butt Muscles Turn Off When We Walk?

Muscles activate when we use the body in a way that recruits them. The gluteal muscles are no different. The two components required to naturally activate gluteal muscles are to 1) unlock the knees when walking and 2) allow the body to move forward with the advancing foot.

Many people lock their knees when they stand or walk. Standing for a couple minutes or longer, most of you will notice you have subconsciously locked one or both of your knees. This conserves energy turning off key leg muscles that hold up the body. Weight bearing is then dispersed through ligaments, **cartilage** (the smooth surface of your joints), **labrum** (tissue that surrounds the hip joint and deepens the socket), and **meniscus** (tissue that helps guide knee joint motions). This tends to break down these structures over time.

While this conserves energy, it turns off the gluteal muscles which are critical to many functions in the lower body system and consequently the pelvis and spine. One reason knee-locking happens while walking is because most shoes have large, padded heels which allow the advancing leg to swing forward in front of the person and strike that heel on the hard ground firmly. This causes the knee to lock immediately upon impact which then turns off the gluteal muscles. They remain quiet until the body catches up to, and passes over, that foot which is too late to control the pelvis and leg adequately, damaging the lower body, pelvis and back.

To test this theory, walk on hard concrete outside for one block with bare feet and you will notice a subtle shift in your walking pattern. The advancing heel no longer strikes the ground quite as hard and perhaps the stride length has shortened, and the knee has become softer. This creates an environment in which the gluteals then can naturally activate. Tiptoe and ice-skate walking corrects this pattern, turning on the gluteals immediately and naturally.

Knee Taping 📹

Because this is a subconscious habit that is driven by locking the knees, it is helpful to create a reminder to keep the knees unlocked. I have developed a simple taping technique that helps with this (Note: knee taping is also featured in Chapter 6).

Simply stand with your knees bent slightly. Place one strip of athletic tape, about 10–12 inches long, on the backs of your knees so that it ends equally above and below the knee joints (Figure 11.5).

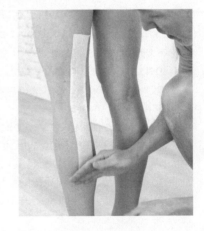

Figure 11.5 Knee taping can quickly train the brain and body to unlock knees to help turn on gluteal muscles.

When you stand up from this position and try to lock your knees, you will now feel the tug of the tape reminding you to keep them unlocked. Because strong tape is needed for this, I use CoverRoll Stretch tape together with Leukotape P. Both can be found on Amazon. A link to this tape, as well as videos of exercises and tests found in this book, can be found on www.rickolderman.com, look under the "Books" tab, and enter the code: PainPatterns.

Initially you will need to shorten your steps to accommodate this new strategy. Gradually your hips and pelvis will learn what is necessary to take longer strides with softer knees—this usually takes about two to three days.

Caution 🖐 The tape I recommend tends to have a high acid content in the adhesive which creates a strong bond with the skin, but this has the potential to irritate the skin. Whenever you remove the tape, ensure that you clean your skin fully. The skin on the backs of the knees is naturally very thin, so my advice to you is the first time you use this tape, please keep it on for between two and four hours maximum, then remove it and inspect your skin for any potential irritation. Use appropriately once you are confident it is causing no major damage to your skin. You may well find that without any noticeable skin reaction, you will be able to wear the tape continuously for up to a week as it is waterproof.

Your Pain Pattern Lesson

Poor walking patterns resulting in deactivation of gluteal muscles accentuate or deepen pain patterns you may have adopted. As a consequence, pelvic orientation is poorly controlled and, if gluteal function is asymmetrical, Side-bending Problems can ensue. Fixing your gait is a critical solution that you could easily miss when addressing pain. The gluteals have multiple functions and activating them naturally will improve many movement and tension problems in the lower body and back system.

Chapter 12   Foot and Ankle Problems

Client Connection

Yuko had suffered from right-sided sciatica for several months. Her injury history had no significant pain or injuries prior to her complaints, and she had not participated in sports or other aggressive recreational activities. Her sciatic pain had apparently appeared out of thin air but caused her to experience terrible pain while sleeping and also for the first few hours after waking. Our Zoom session revealed she had Right Sidebending Problem and Extension Problem patterns which we corrected. In the ensuing three weeks, she dutifully modified her daily activities to counter these problems, as well as corrected asymmetries in her strength and range of motion which were also contributing to them. We made good progress, but she was only 50% better and still could not sleep on her right side—her preferred sleeping position. Clearly, we had missed something important. I watched her bend over (Chapter 13) and noticed a subtle difference in her technique when her right foot was forward compared to when she bent over with her left foot forward. I then tested her calf and soleus range of motion, and we discovered that her right ankle had half the range of motion as her left. When I asked her about this, Yuko had no idea why this might be happening as she had no previous knowledge that there was a problem. The good news is that we successfully managed to address this newly discovered problem using the recommendations in this chapter and the rest of her sciatic pain melted away over the next two weeks. She was finally able to sleep on her right side with no sciatica.

The Foot and Ankle

Our bodies interact with the world through our feet when walking or standing. Consequently, problems with our feet can have a widespread effect up the kinetic chain of events, even potentially contributing to headaches (see Functional Linking in Chapter 5).

To walk correctly, the knee must advance over the foot of the advancing leg easily and at the time of foot strike (Chapter 11). The ease of this motion is primarily governed by the length or tension of the calf and soleus muscles. These collectively blend to form the Achilles tendon which attaches to the heel bone and is continuous with the plantar fascia on the bottom of the foot. Resistance here has two potential consequences:

1. Excessive force is driven into the arch and bones of the foot, stressing those tissues, including the plantar fascia, heel bones or other joints, even contributing to bunions.

2. Excessive force moves upward to the knee, preventing it from bending adequately and contributing to knee-locking (Chapters 6 and 11). This then potentially contributes to other problems at the hip, SI joint, pelvis, back, and rib cage.

Foot Arch Flattening Due to Calf Tightness

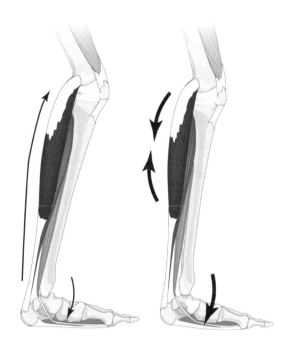

Figure 12.1 Decreased length or increased tension in the calf and/or soleus muscles can increase forces driven into various foot tissues.

These responses can be either unilateral or bilateral. Often when changes in pain do not happen rapidly enough, or if there is a leveling-off of benefits, tightness or problems in the calf and soleus muscles are usually to blame.

Ankle Motion Testing 🎥

Calf Length Test

Step 1.
Place a 2-inch thick book on the ground against a wall. Place the ball of your left foot on the book while your left heel is on the floor. Be sure that the front of your pelvis is facing the wall in front of you and is not twisted. The right foot will remain behind you in whatever position is comfortable.

Step 2.
Lock your left knee backwards or straight (Figure 12.2).

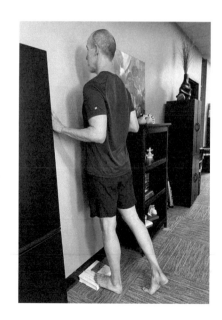

Figure 12.2 Calf length test.

Step 3.
Maintain the locked, backward or straight left knee while bringing your lower body, pelvis, and trunk forward towards the wall. The left heel must remain firmly planted on the floor while doing this and the pelvis must remain facing the wall in front of you. You may use your hands on the wall for balance. Note the tightness you feel in your left calf muscle towards the top of your lower leg and the distance you can move forward towards the wall.

Step 4.
Repeat with the right foot.

Your Results	*Select your answer below*
	✎. __ *My pain is on the right/left (circle one) side of my body.*
	✎. __ *My pain is on both sides of my body.*
	Mark your answers below to the calf length test.
	✎. __ *My right/left (circle one) calf felt tighter than my other calf and it was difficult to lean forward during this test.*
	✎. __ *My tighter side felt about __% tighter than my looser side.*
	✎. __ *Both calves felt equally tight, and it was difficult to lean forward during this test.*
	✎. __ *Neither calf felt tight, and it was easy to lean forward during this test.*

Soleus Length Test

Step 1.
Use the same book as you did for the calf test above and keep it on the ground against the wall. Place the ball of your left foot on the book while your left heel is on the floor as in the calf test above. Be sure that the front of your pelvis is facing the wall in front of you, and it is not twisted. The right foot will remain behind you in whatever position is comfortable.

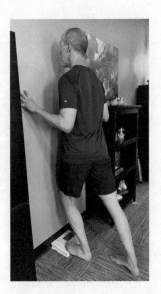

Figure 12.3 Soleus length test.

Step 2.

Bend your left knee towards the wall so that the left knee travels over the second toe of the left foot. The left heel must remain firmly planted on the floor while doing this and the pelvis must remain facing the wall in front of you. You may rest your hands against the wall for balance. Note the tightness you feel in your left soleus muscle, which will be felt towards the bottom of your lower leg closer to your ankle than with the calf test, and the distance you can move forward toward the wall (Figure 12.3).

Step 3.

Repeat with the right foot.

Your Results	*Select your answer below*
	✎ __ *My right/left (circle one) soleus felt tighter than my other soleus and my knee was not able to move forward over my right toes or it was difficult to move it forward.*
	✎ __ *My tighter side felt about __% tighter than my looser side.*
	✎ __ *Both sides felt equally tight, and it was difficult to move forward during this test.*
	✎ __ *Neither side felt tight, and it was easy to move forward during this test.*

Interpreting Your Results 🎥

Tightness, restrictions, or tension in the calf and/or soleus muscles could be caused by older, forgotten injuries—anything from ankle sprains to foot fractures. Tightness in these tissues often comes as a surprise to many of you. I believe this is the case because there are so many different ways to compensate for loss of range of motion at the ankle.

Clinically, I found that the calf and soleus stretches offered in clinics or via the internet, while helpful, rarely if ever solve this problem, primarily because the problem is directly related to our sleep habits.

It seems the cause of tightness in these muscles is due to how we sleep. Most of you will create plantarflexion when side-lying while sleeping by actively pointing your toes away from you, or when lying on your back with the covers lying on your feet or if lying on your stomach, the bed then causes this to happen. The foot and ankle remain in this position for 6–9 hours, shortening the calf and soleus muscles.

To solve this problem, I will ask you to wear a dorsal night splint (Figure 12.4), which is essentially an ankle brace that keeps the foot in a neutral position while sleeping. This simple device became a miracle cure for everything from plantar fasciitis to sciatic or back pain,

depending on whether the testing came back positive for tightness in the calf or soleus muscles. Of course, this worked because we also fixed the other systemic problems further up the legs such as walking (Chapter 11) or other habits associated with pain.

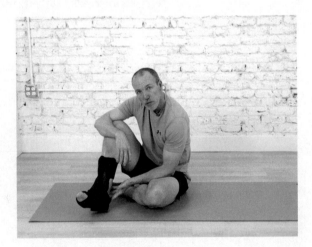

Figure 12.4 A dorsal night splint will help correct tight or tense calf and/or soleus muscles.

Clinical Pearl

For those of you who actively contract your calf or soleus muscles at night, wearing a dorsal night splint will be painful or very irritating. Essentially those muscles are performing an isometric contraction (a sustained contraction where the joint angle does not change) against the night splint for many hours while you sleep. To avoid this pain, instead put the night splint on after going to the bathroom in the middle of the night. This will bestow the benefits of the splint when first waking up and taking the first steps of the morning. Gradually increase wear time as able. The goal will be to wear the night splint through the night with no irritation. At that point, you should re-test the calf and soleus muscles above to see what effect this has had on your ankle motion.

Your Pain Pattern Lesson

Asymmetry in the tightness of calf and soleus muscles can contribute to Sidebending Problems, hip, knee or foot problems. Tightness may be on the same side of the Sidebending Problem or on the opposite side, contributing to a compensation pattern (Chapter 8). Symmetrical calf and soleus tightness will also contribute to an Extension Problem, due to their role in promoting knee-locking and therefore poor gluteal activation and anterior pelvic tilt. Especially since the ankle and foot are far away from the back and pelvis, many practitioners fail to link sources of problems here to problems further up the kinetic chain.

Chapter 13 Bending

Client Connection

Sandy suffered from back pain for years. We discovered she had a Sidebending Problem and Extension Problem and we had made very good progress correcting the tight or weak muscles and walking habits that fed her pain patterns. But her pain persisted—especially during common household chores, like washing dishes and vacuuming. This was a sign that we had not addressed all the habits feeding her pain patterns. I asked her to pretend that she was at the kitchen sink and observed her method of cleaning dishes. I then pulled out our clinic vacuum cleaner and asked her to show me how she vacuumed. I discovered that she used an Extension Problem strategy to perform these tasks by locking her low back into an arched position at all times. After teaching her to relax her spine and change her foot position, she could perform these and other chores without experiencing any pain.

Bending Down

Thus far, with the exception of walking, we have looked at tests that identify tight or weak muscles that contribute to the three primary patterns of pain. Just as important are daily movement habits that reinforce these patterns.

Bending over to brush our teeth or to clean dishes at a sink are two frequent behaviors that can cause significant pain in many of you who suffer from low back or sciatic pain. You will test your preferred method of movement during this common task to gain insight into your pain patterns. You can then apply this information to any bending behaviors such as sitting down or standing up from a chair, or picking objects up off the floor.

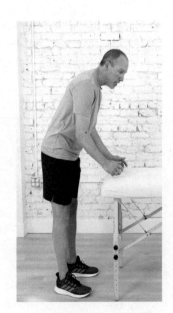

Figure 13.1 Bending test.

Bending Test

Stand at your kitchen or bathroom sink and bend slightly forward to turn on the water, return to an upright position, then bend forward to turn it off again (Figure 13.1).

✋ **Please do not read further until you've performed this test and marked your answers on page 95.** It would be more beneficial to video record this task on your phone to study more closely.

Your Results | *Select your answer below regarding your foot position during the bending test*

✎. __ *My feet were arranged in parallel, side by side, roughly shoulder width apart.*

✎. __ *My feet were staggered with my left/right (circle one) foot slightly forward and the other foot further back, roughly shoulder width apart.*

Mark one of the answers below regarding your low back.

✎. __ *My low back remained erect and relatively rigid as I bent forward and when returning to an upright position.*

✎. __ *My low back flexed or was bent with less of an arch as I bent forward and when returning to an upright position.*

Interpreting Your Results 🎥

Foot Position

In my clinical experience, 99% of you who experience low back or sciatic pain have an Extension Problem as a primary pattern contributing to your pain (Chapter 6). Most of you stand with your feet positioned in parallel (side by side) when bending forward. This contributes to knee-locking and consequently poor butt muscle activation, excessive arching of the lower spine together with focused hinging at the L5/S1 junction (Extension Problems). If you stand like this, your body is predisposed to stand or move with an Extension Problem pattern. This becomes more pronounced when returning from a bent-over position—which is when most people experience pain while bending.

Staggering the feet so that one is forward and one further back and then shifting weight onto the forward leg, helps unlock the Extension Problem pattern, relieving pain, especially when allowing the low back to soften and bend a little rather than remain rigidly arched. The forward leg can then absorb more stress by bending the knee to lower you down and help you stand back up while straightening. This removes extension stress from the L5/S1 junction.

Bending to the Floor

This technique can also be applied to picking lightweight objects up off the floor. Allowing the spine to relax while bending down and placing more emphasis on the forward leg should actually feel good for the back, if you have an Extension Problem. Maintaining that relaxed spine for as long as possible when returning to upright standing will disperse forces throughout the spinal column and legs, reducing pain. This is the technique that helped Jim, mentioned in the Introduction of this book.

For those of you with Flexion Problems the reverse would be true. You will need to maintain an arched spine while bending forward and returning to an upright position.

Your Pain Pattern Lesson

We subconsciously tap into our pain pattern behaviors during most daily activities, such as bending over to turn on the faucet and then returning to an upright position. Taking time to break down and evaluate your most painful activities with a pain-pattern filter will help reveal those hidden behaviors that contribute to your pain. Recording a video on your phone can be very illuminating for this purpose.

Most of you will discover that you are extending your spine to return to an upright position rather than using your legs. This contributes to an Extension Problem pattern. If one leg is used more than the other, then this becomes a Sidebending Problem pattern. Experimenting with these techniques will reveal improved ways of approaching those common activities. Often patients have surprised me with their own novel methods to reverse these patterns.

Chapter 14   Testing for Neck Pain and Headaches

Client Connection

Rachel lived on a ranch and suffered chronic migraine headaches, neck pain and had neural radicular symptoms into both hands. Her MRI revealed many changes in her neck bones and/or soft tissues. She was scheduled for a third cortisone shot in three weeks. The first two resulted in temporary improvement of about 50% pain reduction, however their usefulness quickly faded. Through using the Armpit Test below, we determined that her pain came from her shoulder blades. Rachel's neck pain, headaches, and radicular symptoms rapidly reduced by correcting the muscles that pulled her shoulder blades down and her postural patterns that contributed to this problem.

Neck Pain & Headaches

Chronic tension and pain apply to the top of our spinal column too. In fact, when we think of tension, one of the first images that comes to mind is of someone scrunching up their face and shrugging their shoulders—the Startle Reflex pattern.

Similar to the lumbar spine, pain in the cervical (neck) spine will commonly have diagnoses like herniated discs, arthritic changes, or stenosis, all of which create radicular (radiating) symptoms down the arm, or headaches. Similar to sciatica, all the blame is traditionally placed on the vertebrae in the spine or the discs between them, as if these problems emerged spontaneously, without provocation. While it is

true that cervical bony structures can impinge the nerve roots or irritate the neck or head, now you can see that there are likely other systemic issues which can contribute to the formation of those structural changes in the neck, causing irritation.

Another biomechanical stressor to this system, outside of the fascial patterns identified earlier, are the shoulder blades (**scapulae**) which rest on top of the rib cage. Typically, the shoulder blades become **depressed**, by which I mean that they sit too low on the rib cage or that there are too many forces trying to pull them lower down toward the pelvis.

For a deeper dive into my approach to solving chronic neck pain and headaches, please refer to my book, *Fixing You®: Neck Pain & Headaches* (Boone Publishing, 2009). A link to this book can be found at www.rickolderman.com, then simply click the "Books" tab. For more current interventions use my digital home program also found at www.rickolderman.com and then click the "Fixing You® Programs" tab.

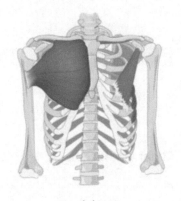

(a)

There are many reasons for this, primary among them is a faulty posture strategy that activates scapular depressor muscles (Figure 14.1a and 14.1b), pulling the shoulder blades down.

(b)

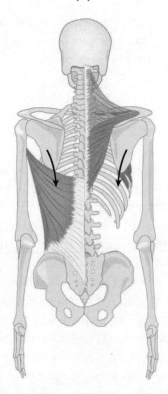

Figure 14.1 Upper body muscles in the front of the trunk (a) and the back of the trunk (b) that contribute to scapular depression.

Certain sports or exercise programs emphasize this behavior, such as dance, gymnastics, yoga and Pilates. These activities promote a "long neck", together with an erect spine. Cues to achieve these aesthetic qualities are framed with instructions, such as "Bring your shoulder blades together and down into your back pockets," or "Squeeze your shoulder blades together," or something along those lines. This is a faulty posture strategy, perpetuating scapular depression and consequently chronic shoulder, neck, and headache pain.

There are significant muscular/fascial connections from the shoulder blades to the neck bones and base of the skull which then create excessive tension and forces absorbed by these spinal structures (Figure 14.2).

I devised a simple test that will help you establish if your shoulder blades are contributing to your chronic neck pain or headaches—the Armpit Test.

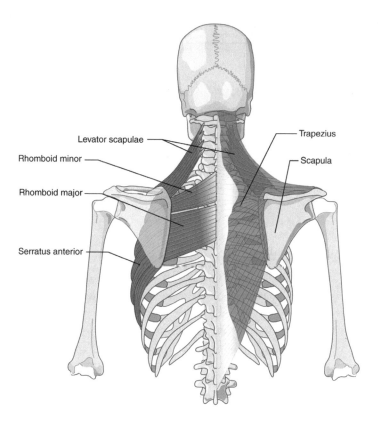

Figure 14.2 The shoulder blades have many muscular connections into the cervical spine and skull potentially creating neck pain and headaches.

The Armpit Test 📹

Your Results	Select your answer below
	✎ __ I have a Sidebending Problem on my left/right (circle one) side.
	✎ __ My neck/shoulder/headache pain is primarily on my left/right/ (circle one) side.
	✎ __ My neck/shoulder/headache pain is primarily central.

For this test, you will need some assistance.

Step 1.

Begin by moving your head around to test your pain. Turn your head left and right to look over your shoulders, look up and down and note at what point in your movements you experience pain or restrictions. Rate that pain on a 0–10 scale (0 = no pain, 10 = emergency room pain).

Be precise in your assessment by also noting the amount of movement that triggers pain. For instance, "Turning my head 30 degrees to the left creates 7/10 pain". Record your pain and movement notes below:

Your Results	*Select your answer below*
	✎. __ *I have pain turning my head Left/Right/Both (circle one).* *Notes (such as range of motion, difficulty turning, restrictions, etc.)*
	✎. __ *I have pain looking Up/Down/Both (circle one).* *Notes (such as range of motion, difficulty moving the head, restrictions, etc.)*
	✎. __ *My pain is a __ when I do these movements (0–10).* *Notes (such as the range of motion triggering pain, whether you are able to move through it, etc.)*

Step 2.

Your helper will now stand behind you and place their hands in your armpits. They will then lift your shoulders up about an inch higher than normal (Figure 14.3). Your job is to completely relax your shoulders and let them lift 100% of your shoulder system weight. Your shoulder system can weigh between 15–40 pounds—more if you are actively contracting shoulder depressor muscles—so your helper should be strong enough to hold this system up for about 30–60 seconds.

For many of you, it can be difficult to relax your shoulders. In that case your helper may need to slowly jiggle your shoulders a little, to help you relax.

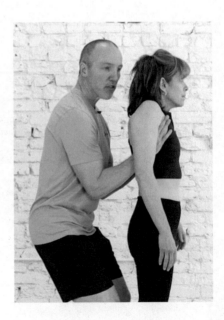

Figure 14.3 The Armpit Test involves a helper passively lifting your shoulder system higher to unload muscular connections between the shoulder blade and the neck and head.

Once you are completely relaxed, and your helper continues to hold your shoulders up, move your head around and note any increase in range of motion or a sense of reduction of tension or pain. (Note, have your helper observe as well. I have often found that many of you are unable to notice changes in range of motion as a result of this test, even though I can see a significant difference!) Compare this to your initial notes (above) about your pain.

Note: The nerves that feed your arms and hands travel through the armpit area. So, when your helper is holding your shoulder system up, they will be pressing on those nerves. In such an event, you will likely feel radicular symptoms in your hands during this test, especially if you have already been suffering from radicular symptoms.

This is normal and should' not be confused with assessing your head and neck range of motion or pain during those movements. When your helper removes their hands, those symptoms will dissipate again.

Step 3.

After you have assessed the change in your range of motion and pain, your helper should then gently lower your shoulders back down. At this point your shoulder girdle system should now be fully returned to your body and you may feel the weight of this system on your upper body more precisely, which may mean a return of pain. How quickly your pain returns is an indication of how significant the downward forces are on your shoulder blades.

Your Results   *Select your answer below*

✎. __ *My pain reduced by (or my range of motion improved by) __% while my shoulders were held higher. Or, I felt increased tension or pain once my shoulders were lowered back down. This indicates that my shoulder blades are a significant source of my tension and pain.*

✎. __ *My pain was not reduced while my shoulders were held higher. This is unusual for those of you with chronic neck pain and headaches. Please re-test to confirm. Be sure you are truly relaxing your shoulder system onto the hands of your helper.*

Most of you will feel a sense of relief or reduction in pain during this test which confirms that your shoulder blades are having a significant effect on your pain. Please understand that, if you have been diagnosed with structural changes mentioned above and have been told those are the sources of your pain, you now understand that the shoulder blades are acting on those sources, causing them to be problematic. We have not changed those structures. Instead, we have changed the forces acting on them, a primary irritant being the shoulder blade system.

Fix Depressed Shoulder Blades

All-Fours Rocking 📹

Begin in a hands-and-knees position with your hands under your shoulders and knees under your hips. Be sure that your lower back is flat by drawing your belly button in towards your spine. Exhale and rock back onto your feet while anchoring your hands in their starting position (Figure 14.4).

Feel that the floor is pulling your arms into an overhead position as you rock back on your heels. Allow your shoulders to passively shrug up toward your ears. Be sure the back of your neck, especially at the base of the skull, remains lengthened and even rest your head on a pillow, if necessary. Feel a nice stretch through the shoulder blade or armpit area. Feel free to slide your hands forward on the floor, if you'd like to feel more stretch. Return to the starting position after holding at the bottom for five breaths. Perform 3–5 repetitions. Alternatively, this can be done sitting at a dining room table and/or walking both hands to either side to further stretch the rib cage. Perform this routine several times a day to reduce the downward pull of your shoulder blades.

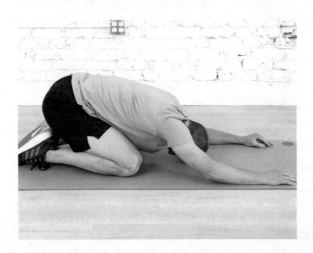
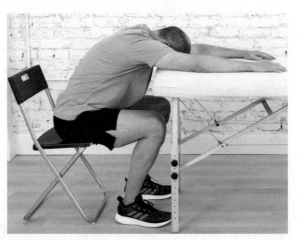

Figure 14.4 All Fours Rocking Stretch lengthens scapular depressor muscles.

Lifting the Rib Cage 📹

As mentioned earlier, those of you with depressed shoulder blades have typically developed a faulty posture pattern whereby you are pinching your shoulders together to create an erect posture or a long neck (this also contributes to an Extension Problem). The shoulder blades rest outside of the rib cage and are not meant to be the prime generators of posture. Using the Lifting the Rib Cage exercise will help you to correct this posture strategy by teaching you to use your core muscles to achieve good posture instead.

Refer to Chapter 6 for an explanation on how to perform Lifting the Rib Cage.

Your Pain Pattern Lesson

Depressed shoulder blades are one of the most commonly missed problems leading to chronic upper body, neck and head pain, even in the case of radiating symptoms down the arms. Stretching the muscles that are depressing the shoulder blades is a strong first step to solving this type of pain. A primary postural habit that creates shoulder blade depression is that of bringing the shoulder blades down and back into the back pockets or squeezing them together to assist with creating an erect posture—this essentially contributes to an Extension Problem. Using the Lifting the Rib Cage strategy in the Flexion Problem solutions (Chapter 6) is a great way to retrain posture strategies.

For more stories about how this information solved difficult neck pain and headache cases and other interesting cases, please read my book *Solving the Pain Puzzle: Cases from 25 Years as a Physical Therapist* (McFarland, 2023).

If neck pain or headaches are unilateral, this may be due to a Sidebending Problem with a lowered rib cage on the side of the scapular depression helping to pull down that shoulder blade (Please review your answers above to confirm this connection). Remember the shoulder blade rests on the rib cage. This may be confirmed if you walked your hands side-to-side during the All Fours Rocking exercise and found your rib cage to be tighter on the same side of your neck pain or headaches. Performing the Reaching While Walking correction found in Chapter 7 can also help with this problem.

This unilateral pain may also be due to older injuries on the same side of your upper body. Chapter 19 will help you review these old injuries.

Chapter 15 Your Brain Bias

Client Connection

Nevell had suffered from chronic back pain for the last three years. We discovered this was due to his faulty walking pattern, together with his retroverted femurs, and I was able to teach him to walk correctly (Chapters 11 and 10, respectively). Initially, he resisted this change because it was so different from how he had become so used to walking. We showed him, however, that walking correctly immediately reduced his pain. This helped him re-frame his judgments about walking differently. Within three weeks of mastering a better gait, his back pain disappeared completely.

Brain Bias

You have learned in Chapter 4 how the brain monitors sensations and creates motor output to negotiate our daily life and create muscle tone and tension. A large part of that output includes programs stored in our cerebellum that help us perform commonly repeated tasks like walking, postural control, sitting, or washing dishes, etc., so we can efficiently go about our day without having to re-learn from scratch how to perform these tasks.

But now you are gaining insight into the fact that how you have been performing those tasks has probably been corrosive to your body over time and has played a big role in your current pain by feeding into these primary pain patterns. This next test will show you clearly how your brain's messages are helping or harming your attempts to solve your pain.

The Hand-Clasping Test 🎥

Clasp your hands together with interlocking fingers, as if praying (Figure 15.1). Look down and notice which thumb and fingers are on top of

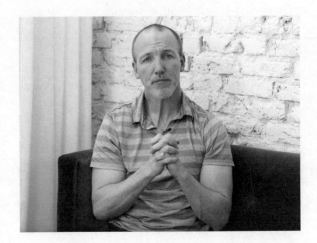

Figure 15.1 Clasp hands together.

the others. Take a few seconds to see how this feels to you. It should feel natural and easy. You probably did not even need to look down at your hands to clasp them together.

Now unclasp your hands and, without looking, re-clasp them together *but this time with the opposite thumb and fingers on top.* You may have peeked to make sure you were doing it right (or at least wanted to). Now look down and check your work. How did you do? Keep your hands clasped together in this way while reading the rest of this chapter.

Notice how this feels. Your cerebellum, which holds your habitual pattern for hand clasping, is telling your cerebral cortex that this is not how things are typically done. There are other parts of your brain that have judged this different feeling as "wrong" and therefore it must be "bad" for you. They may even be creating an emotional response, such as frustration or irritation. Your cerebral cortex is overriding these concerns for the moment even though this feels a little annoying to you. It realizes this is just a simple test and so you're going to hang in there a little while longer, in spite of all these alerts.

What does this test tell us about pain or tension? Well, you just learned that habits are programmed in your cerebellum. We also know that the body can heal just about anything in approximately three months. However, because you are experiencing chronic pain, something about your hidden habits must be hurting you. You are not consciously aware of this though (remember that your brain is wired for short-term success, not figuring out what habits might be hurting you). From this moment forward, even if you were to change those habits to solve your pain, your brain will set off alarms, alerting you that something is different. Parts of your brain will likely judge those changes as "wrong"

or "bad", similar to those feelings you have just experienced.

But your conscious self does not really *know* if these changes are wrong or bad. Similar to clasping your hands differently, it simply was not what you were used to. This test shows you that different does not necessarily mean "bad." In fact, where changing pain-causing habits is concerned, different may very well mean "good."

I have detailed this test and explanation because, as you learn to change how you use your body, you will meet resistance—from the inside, like Nevell above. You must have the patience to discover whether what you are attempting is beneficial or not rather than whether or not it is familiar. This will be more difficult than you can imagine, and you must be ready to objectively judge your future attempts to solve your tension and pain. Remember about the brain in Chapter 4, where we learned that we can change that motor map of our body, the homunculus, in our motor cortex? This is your opportunity to do just that.

It will be very easy to slip into your old movement patterns, so setting up external reminders will help cue you to check in on yourself when trying to change these painful behaviors. I recommend wearing a watch or bracelet on the wrong wrist. This annoys most people, causing them to frequently notice it. Each time they notice it is an opportunity to check in on some behavior they are trying to change. If there are certain tasks that trigger your pain pattern, such as brushing your teeth at the sink, then perhaps place garage sale stickers on implements associated with that task (such as the sink faucet or mirror in this case) to remind you to take a moment and move more slowly and more constructively to unravel your pain.

Your Pain Pattern Lesson

Fixing chronic pain will necessarily involve doing things differently than you are used to. Your old ways of using your body are what contribute to your current pain by reinforcing your pain patterns. Re-framing brain alerts to replace judgment with objective observation will help you rapidly adopt better movement habits that will lead to a decrease in your pain.

Chapter 16 Practical Application
Lisa's Sciatic Pain

Lisa, a recent patient in her late thirties, complained that she had experienced left sciatic pain with each of her four pregnancies over the previous seven years. It lingered longer and longer after each pregnancy but would always go away. Now, after her fourth pregnancy, her sciatic pain had not subsided.

During pregnancy, as the fetus grows, a woman will lean back more to offset the forward pull on her pelvis and lower back—this creates an Extension Problem which we confirmed using the test in Chapter 6 (Figure 16.1).

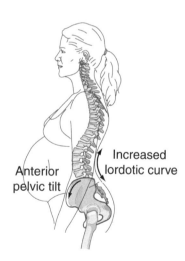

Anterior pelvic tilt

Increased lordotic curve

Figure 16.1 Pregnancy typically creates Extension Problems.

The pattern of her left-sided sciatica lingering longer with each pregnancy indicated to me that she had a potential Left Sidebending

Problem that seemed to be worsening with each pregnancy. I saw her via Zoom and confirmed this using the first Sidebending Test from Chapter 7. She definitely had a larger crease on her left waist that no one had noticed before.

Why would the sciatica go away between pregnancies though? The logical explanation was that in her case, this was a progressively deteriorating condition. In my experience, things that become progressively worse can also become progressively better. The fact that her sciatic pain had resolved between pregnancies showed that she still had resources, but they had slowly deteriorated and eventually broken down completely. To really solve her pain puzzle, I needed to understand *why* these systems were struggling.

I queried her about any history of old injuries—she insisted she had none. This is typical because you are not trained to functionally link old injuries or problems—especially those that no longer cause pain—with current pain. Her body, however, told me a different story. Lisa must have had an older problem which remained hidden until she had more significant and sustained challenges to her system—her pregnancies. Her successive pregnancies deepened the original pattern set up long ago. Each time, she recovered less and less. While we could correct her Extension and Sidebending Problems, we needed to also understand what that original issue was, so these current issues did not return.

After some pestering and standing firm in my conviction, she finally remembered an old ankle injury she had sustained when backpacking 25 years earlier. This was a long, arduous hiking trip with a heavy pack carried over the course of several weeks. Initially she could barely put weight on that injured foot. Her group had to carry her pack for her. As the trip wore on, her pain gradually lessened to the point where she could carry some of her pack weight again. Many weeks after her hike, her pain eventually went away, and she declined to have a medical follow-up. It was so long ago, and in her mind so insignificant that she could not remember which ankle it was.

So, I asked her to perform the Single Leg Standing test (Chapter 8) to determine which ankle was likely injured. Even though she had left sciatica and a Left Sidebending Problem, she chose to stand up from her chair using her left leg first. This made no apparent sense—why would anyone use their painful and injured side first when standing up during this test? Because subconsciously her cerebellum and cerebral cortex had been conditioned to believe that *her left leg* would be able to achieve the desired outcome more successfully. The significance of this meant that her left leg compensated for a right leg problem. Were this not the case, she would have used her non-painful right leg first when she tried to stand up.

Furthermore, she was shocked to learn that her right leg felt 50% weaker than her left leg, even though she worked out with weights under the guidance of a trainer and had a strict cardio regimen. This simple test gave her a conscious understanding of a subconscious pattern of problems stemming from an old ankle sprain 25 years earlier. Her left leg had been carrying an extra 50% of the load all the years since. Finally, her body was telling her, "Look, I've been doing this long enough. And now you've been adding these pregnancies on top of it all! You've got to figure something out here!" That's what chronic tension and pain are—signals that something is wrong now—even if the problems stemmed from long ago. Unfortunately, she was not able to interpret her body's messages until now.

We also explored femoral anteversion and retroversion (Chapter 10)—a new concept for her in spite of the many years she spent seeking medical help for this problem. It turned out that her left femur was anteverted, meaning that her left thigh bone rotated inwards a little too much. In these cases, the thigh bone must be controlled more precisely to avoid excessive internal rotation—the knee and hip joints do not like excessive internal rotation, as this creates increased compression and shear forces in those joints. You have already learned that the gluteus maximus is the primary muscle that controls thigh bone internal rotation.

The gluteus maximus is one of the most powerful muscles in the body and should naturally turn on when we walk. Her gluteal muscles were not turning on. Why? Because as she gained weight during each pregnancy, she locked her knees straight so her leg muscles would not become fatigued. Locking the knees turns off key lower body muscles which have multiple functions, the gluteus maximus being the primary one. It also deepens established pain patterns—in her case, Extension and Left Sidebending Problems. So, she had a left leg that was carrying upwards of a 50% greater load than her right leg and the primary controller of her left anteverted thigh bone, the gluteus maximus, was not turning on when she walked.

Summarizing what we found during Lisa's initial evaluation:

1.	Extension Problem (Chapters 2 and 6)
2.	Left Sidebending Problem (Chapters 4 and 7)
3.	Poor gluteal activity during walking (Chapter 11)
4.	Left thigh muscles tighter than those on her right side (Chapter 9)
5.	Left Anteverted femur (Chapter 10)
6.	Right leg weaker than her left leg (Chapter 8)
7.	Right calf/soleus tighter than her left (Chapter 12)

The mystery and frustration she had been wrestling with for eight years was unveiled in about 15 minutes using the tests and thinking you will find in this book. Her sciatic pain had become progressively more problematic over the years, but her left leg had accepted a significant (over) load long before that—probably since that initial right ankle sprain more than two decades earlier.

It is likely that her brain initially registered the change in gait pattern due to the sprain, similar to clasping your hands differently in Chapter 15. But her brain became habituated to this change because to revert back to her normal walking pattern would have caused intense pain. As the right ankle healed, she could place more weight on it. Her brain no longer had an objective comparison between the two legs to judge just *how much load* she should return to her right leg. Her brain was primarily interested in whether she could walk again without pain to complete

that hiking trip (success-oriented), not *how* she was walking again.

As her left leg worked harder, her cerebellum re-wired in order for her left leg to accept more load than the right leg. Eventually it became a habit with no further need to communicate with her cerebral cortex. As the left leg and waist muscles worked harder and longer, remaining more contracted, muscle spindles likely adjusted to this new length and tension relationship, setting a higher degree of muscle tension in that side of her body (Chapters 4 and 5). Again, because her brain had become habituated to this tension pattern, there were no alarms that sounded as a result—actually that excessive tension was necessary because of how she was loading her left leg. I believe that this is essentially how old injuries or problems can so frequently be connected to current chronic tension and pain.

Her home program to resolve the issue consisted of:

1.	Thigh stretches, with the goal of creating symmetry between the legs and a normal range of motion (Chapter 9)
2.	Reaching While Walking during her first few steps, getting up from seated positions to reprogram her Sidebending Problem (Chapter 7)
3.	Butt Pumps to strengthen her gluteals to improve control of her anteverted femur (Chapter 10)
4.	Paying attention to (and changing) her habit of unloading the right leg in favor of the left (Chapter 14)
5.	Unlocking her knees when standing and walking to remove Extension Problem stress to her spine and to turn on her gluteal muscles naturally (Chapters 6 and 11)
6.	Wearing a dorsal night splint on her right foot several few weeks (Chapter 12)

I also gave her the three somatic lessons, which are featured toward the end of this book (Chapter 21), to reduce tension along her two pain patterns (Extension Problem and Sidebending Problem), as well as to unlock dysfunctional gait patterns that had become her norm.

I showed her how her compensation patterns had been worked into her daily routine, from standing and sitting to turning or bending over (Chapter 13). Once her cerebral cortex was given a new standard by which to compare her current movements, she was able to correct all the habits feeding the asymmetrical usage patterns that she had developed over the last 25 years. The most important habit to change was her walking pattern. We used the information in Chapter 10 to fix those problems.

Her sciatic pain decreased by 50% over the next couple of days, after which we had one more short session to fine-tune her gluteal muscle activation while walking (see Tiptoe Walking in Chapter 11).

Fixing walking patterns is critical to solving most lower body and back pain because walking is the one habit that we engage with most often. It also seems to be the most misunderstood activity we perform, judging by all the books and medical research surrounding walking patterns. Problems here magnify compensation patterns due to frequency and load. Again, changing Lisa's gait set off alarms in her cerebral cortex and cerebellum because she was changing a fundamental movement pattern (Chapter 15). However, this time her cerebral cortex could override these alarms, like maintaining that new hand-clasping pattern we tried earlier, because she understood logically that this was not a "bad" thing, but instead a healing action.

Once she fixed those older issues and gait compensations, her pain completely disappeared over a period approaching three weeks. A follow-up call with her six months later revealed she still had no pain.

This case nicely incorporates all the elements of tension and pain presented in this book. It is by no means unique in that regard. Just about every chronic pain patient I work with goes through a similar process, with similar results. As one of my therapists trained in this approach described it, "It's simpler but more comprehensive." Often my patients don't understand why they feel so much better because they haven't really done anything to get better or to maintain their pain-free status. This is because they have normalized their changes, and their brain is no longer receiving alerts that something has changed.

In other words, they are using their bodies in a manner which causes the fewest tensions and stresses and that actually feeds the body rather than breaking it down.

Your Pain Pattern Lesson

Seeing pain as patterns of problems helps simplify what the sources of the pain are, even though their scope is larger. Because the body works as a system, small changes in one place, like unlocking knees, will have large ripple effects up and down the kinetic chain of events affecting pain patterns.

Chapter 17   Practical Application
Brian's One-Sided Back Pain

Brian was a very athletic, active man in his late 50s who had suffered from right-sided back pain for over 20 years. He went through discectomy surgery (removal of a portion of a herniated disc) about ten years earlier, while also having several cortisone shots, together with multiple practitioners attempting to solve his pain. Nothing helped long-term.

At his initial examination, I identified:

1.	Extension Problem (Chapters 2 & 6)
2.	Right Sidebending Problem (Chapters 4 & 7)
3.	Poor gluteal activity during walking (Chapter 11)
4.	Right thigh muscles tighter than his left thigh muscles (Chapter 9)
5.	Retroverted femurs (Chapter 10)
6.	Symmetrical leg strength (Chapter 8)

For the first four problems, we employed the same fixes that helped Lisa's sciatic pain presented in the previous chapter: unlock knees, reaching while walking, tiptoe walking, butt pumps, and thigh stretches. Because Brian had retroverted femurs, I asked him to begin walking with his feet slightly turned outward for the next week (Chapter 10).

His pain decreased by 75% after that first week, however we were unable to improve beyond that. I recognized that Brian had significant tension throughout his body whenever I tried to move an arm or a leg while he was resting and was met with resistance. So, I employed a neurological technique, Hanna Somatics, to reset muscle spindles in the larger reflex patterns I discussed in Chapter 4.

I decided to target his Sidebending Problem pattern first because his primary complaint was on the right side of his back. Brian was amazed to find he struggled to allow slow, controlled movement of his body—especially when addressing waist and pelvic movements. However, after our first session, he reported that his back pain was 90% reduced. On our next visit, I targeted his Extension Problem pattern of tension. He reported 100% relief for the first time in years. This confirmed neurologically based tension as a significant driver of his pattern of problems.

We continued with these tension-reducing treatments for several weeks, during which time Brian reported that he had no pain. He was completely dumbfounded. As with Lisa, I showed Brian how these pain patterns crept into his everyday activities, and then I taught him alternatives. This would reinforce the pain-reducing changes we'd made up to that point.

Interestingly, several years later I had lunch with Brian—he was still pain free and he could not understand it, because it was effortless for him to remain so even though he had resumed all of his athletic endeavors. He also reported that during our time together, he had been going through a very difficult time in his life and that by simply listening to him, I had helped tremendously. During our sessions he would speak of his personal and professional problems while I released his deeper patterns of tension using Hanna Somatics. It was not until that lunch together that I realized how struggles in his personal life may have been feeding those tension patterns (based on the information in Chapter 3). By talking them out while concurrently releasing the physical expression of those concerns, we had essentially worked on both sides of the coin that created his pain.

Your Pain Pattern Lesson

Psychological tension can often be a hidden problem that locks the body into pain patterns. Paying attention to and writing down thoughts and feelings while addressing pain may help you see connections you were previously unaware of.

Chapter 18 Dietary Sources of Tension

So far, we have only explored the psychological, musculoskeletal, fascial, and brain system roles in creating chronic tension and pain. These include:

1. **Poor movement habits creating tight or weak muscles**
2. **Fascial superhighways containing structures like myofibroblasts sensitive to SNS stimulation through psychological events laid down in mechanically stressed areas**
3. **Activation of ancient large-pattern reflexes**

However, there is one more area that is worth mentioning and which is related to stressors that seem to contribute to chronic tension and pain—dietary sources that include what we can ingest or inhale. These can be foods, allergens, and molds that enter our body and which can cause inflammation that plays out in the musculoskeletal system.

The microbes found in our gut have been linked to anxiety and depression—two conditions that can increase our SNS response and therefore trigger fascial contractions.[44,45]

Gut microbes, referred to as our **gut biome**, have also been linked to rheumatoid arthritis and other joint inflammatory problems.[46]

This is not my area of expertise, but I have heard a sufficient number of stories and seen enough cases to believe that this category of problem should be included here, even though traditional medical research does not seem to address this connection. The following information is my attempt to link dietary issues to musculoskeletal pain.

Celiac Disease

Gluten intolerance can have far-reaching effects on the body. It has been found that up to 50% of people with celiac disease could develop **peripheral neuropathy** (problems with nerve transmission signals from feet or hands) which may even precede the discovery of gluten intolerance.[47, 48, 49]

Correcting walking strategies is very important to solving most lower body, pelvic, and back pain. Solving arm and shoulder blade movements is a big part of fixing upper body, neck, and headache pain. **Ataxia**, which means "without coordination," describes a problem with how you move your body and which can be the result of neurological changes from celiac disease.[50]

Crohn's Disease

Crohn's Disease, a type of inflammatory bowel disease, can also cause a reduction in skeletal muscle strength and mass, and also cause fatigue.[51,52,53] As leg muscles weaken and/or energy levels are depleted, people typically begin locking their knees straight when standing and walking. This puts load-bearing stress on joints rather than progressively weakening muscles. However, you now understand that locking the knees turns off the gluteus maximus, which is involved in many roles critical to movement health.

Mold

Lastly, I have only anecdotal evidence of mold causing unusual neurological or musculoskeletal problems in one or two of my patients (*Solving the Pain Puzzle*, McFarland, 2023). Internally generated problems are often the last places medical providers might look, especially given the lack of medical research supporting some of these ideas. Anecdotally though, I have seen a few cases where unexplained pain seemed to have been caused by these factors.

Your Pain Pattern Lesson

The body can respond to internal processes involving digestion or other things we inhale by creating inflammation played out in the musculoskeletal system. The body's response to these problems can fall into the three pain patterns discussed in this book—Extension Problems, Flexion Problems and/or Sidebending Problems.

Chapter 19   The Three Pillars of Pain

Chapters 6-14 should help you identify and solve older, hidden problems that feed into the three primary pain patterns. This chapter will dive a little deeper to complete the whole picture for you.

Go into the self-help or medical section of any bookstore and you will find hundreds of different books trying to help people who are in pain. They all seem to boil down to addressing three types of problems: musculoskeletal, emotional/spiritual/psychological, or dietary/ allergens/mold. This book has been my attempt to bring these three areas together under one roof, so to speak, to explain how these issues can potentially manifest as chronic musculoskeletal tension and pain.

I think of these types of problems as Three Pillars of Pain. We all have a threshold above which we experience pain. There seems to be three primary areas (pillars) that push us up to and beyond that threshold:

1. **Musculoskeletal issues, like tight or weak muscles or problems with biomechanics, fascia, global reflex activation or movement habits.**
2. **Emotional/spiritual/psychological issues that trigger a stress response manifesting in our body via fascia, reflex patterns and which then affect movement habits.**
3. **Dietary/allergens/mold issues causing a global inflammatory or stress response also expressed in our musculoskeletal system via fascia or reflex pattern activation.**

Because we have unique genetics and morphology, brain chemistry, biochemistry, lifestyle, exercise or work habits, injuries, psychological make-up, etc., the composition of those three pillars will be different for each person. So, while these issues create the same three patterns of pain, the compositions of these stressors are unique to the individual.

My focus as a physical therapist is on the musculoskeletal system. The information in this book helps explain why your neighbor's solution to their sciatica may be different from the solution to your sciatica, even if the pain is virtually identical. For instance, an old right ankle injury was the source of Lisa's left sciatic pain (Chapter 16). However, it could just as easily have been a left knee or foot problem, a right hip problem, a retroverted right femur, a traumatic car accident several years ago—any number of issues that then manifests as one or two of the three patterns of pain through a series of compensations. This is then compounded by all those other lifestyle factors (sports played, emotional trauma, etc.) mentioned earlier. Ultimately, whatever the causes of the pain, they are expressed in these same three patterns of problems—Extension, Flexion, and/ or Sidebending. Solving the pattern is fairly simple. Doing detective work to understand *why* the pattern is happening requires more thought, which is what Chapters 6–14 address.

To highlight this, recently an old college friend of mine called me, he was complaining of right-sided back pain. His medical providers told him it was a quadratus lumborum (QL) spasm. As we saw in Chapter 7, the QL attaches from the pelvis to the lumbar spine at varying levels. Because of the unilateral nature of his pain, I immediately suspected a Right Sidebending Problem. I inquired about his past history, and he said that he had no right-sided injuries. I then asked him to perform the single leg standing test from Chapter 8 to see if he was compensating for an older left-side injury. He was not and still denied that there were any right-sided issues after repeated queries.

His right thigh muscles were significantly tighter than his left thigh muscles, so I gave him the thigh stretch (Chapter 9) to get started and asked him to re-establish the thigh muscle symmetry between his two legs. He texted me an hour later to let me know that his right-sided pain already felt much better after his first stretching session. I suspected the thigh tightness was the cause of his pain—but I still did not understand *why* the right thigh muscles were tighter. Later he informed me that he thought the pain was happening because he had not been exercising after his surgery. Surgery?! He had failed to mention this in our call, even after my persistent questions. He then said he'd been treated for prostate cancer last year, and this involved radiation targeting his right side and after which he rested. When he became more active, his pain began. I assume this was

a contributing factor to his right thigh tightness.

I have included this story to show that underlying causes of pain are often off our radar. Even when I asked him directly and repeatedly about *any* right-sided problems, he denied there was any history of injuries. This is because he was not trained to functionally link older or apparently unrelated or obscure problems to his current pain. After all, prostate cancer should not have anything to do with QL pain. And it did not, at least not directly. However, the treatment for it may have. When I explained this to him, it seemed a very obvious connection, given the timing and his activity level.

Being more thoughtful about your pain means dredging up history that would never seem to have anything to do with your pain. I have learned to take people's answers to my questions with a grain of salt because the body does not lie. I eventually uncovered the truth because this information is so reliable, and I understand that pain is the body's way of communicating an immediate problem.

There are myriad structural diagnoses relating to spinal pain, such as disc bulges/herniations, stenosis, spondylolisthesis, degenerative disc disease, arthritic changes, sciatica, radiculopathy, SI joint pain, and more. However, when performing the tests and solutions found in Chapters 6–14, you likely have found that your body was not working quite as well as you thought. If the structural diagnoses listed above were simply to blame for your pain, then pain levels should not change after performing a brief test or exercise. **Therefore, the stresses acting on your spine are as important, if not more so, than the structures blamed for your pain in many cases.** This is another lesson your body is trying to teach you.

Fix the pattern of problems and you will usually fix the pain, no matter how long it has been around or what has shown up on those scans. If you have had surgery and it failed to solve your pain, you now understand why—the system of problems causing your pain (or those structural problems) has never been addressed. The surgeon may have fixed the structures, however the repeated hammering from these subconscious patterns on those vulnerable tissues had not changed.

Yet one of the most common questions I hear as a physical therapist is: "Which exercises will fix my back pain, sciatica, or _____ (insert diagnosis here)?" You now understand that this is not really the right question to ask. My answer is always, "It depends on what the problem is which is causing your pain." Do you have an Extension Problem? Flexion Problem? Sidebending Problem? And then the next question is "Why?" If there were one or two exercises that solved all back or sciatica pain in all people, I think they would have been plastered all over the internet by now and found on handouts in every doctor's or PT's office.

The good news is, as you saw with the cases of Lisa, Brian and the others presented in this book, a chronic problem does not need years to resolve. Nor does it require countless exercises or perpetual office visits. Once you understand the nature of the problem, most issues can be corrected relatively quickly and simply, thanks to our body's amazing ability to heal once obstacles are removed. All you really need is the right information.

Identify Your 3 Pillars of Pain

As with any problem, it helps if you know what the actual cause is. For instance, if you have chronic back pain and have a history of unresolved anxiety, stress, or trauma, then this could be considered a potential stressor for your back (by virtue of fascia containing a high concentration of SNS nerve fibers and myofibroblasts in the low back area—see Chapter 3). All the stretching or core strengthening in the world will not change that psychological pillar pushing you toward your critical pain threshold. Yes, there may be biomechanical issues, however the psychological issues might be primary and the biomechanical issues secondary contributors.

It is important to understand that even if you have all three of these pillars of pain operating, they funnel into the same three chronic patterns of tension—Extension, Flexion, and/or Sidebending—which then causes musculoskeletal pain.

What I have learned, at least in the case of musculoskeletal and emotional issues, is that the funnel works both ways. Solve tension or biomechanical/movement problems and you can begin to change the sources of that tension. In the case of emotionally derived sources of tension, I have found in my patients a calming emotional effect after reducing their musculoskeletal tension and pain. Sometimes as we unravel their pain patterns, memories, dreams, or flashes of insight occur that often point to the psychological or dietary source of their problems. They just need to be attentive to these messages and not dismiss them.

So, the first step in solving chronic tension and pain would be to identify where your pain is.

Please record your responses below:

1. ✎ __ Describe the pain you are trying to solve. Please be specific.

a.	Where is it located?
b.	Left, right or both sides?
c.	Is there an activity such as walking, sitting, bending etc., that triggers your pain consistently?
d.	Describe the above activity, including time, repetitions, movements, or other elements associated with triggering that pain that help quantify it. Perhaps even make a video of yourself performing that activity. This may give you an objective view of what is going on.
e.	What is your pain level on a scale of 0–10 (0=no pain, 10=worst imaginable pain) when performing this activity?
f.	When did your pain begin?
g.	Was it triggered by an accident or other physical or emotional trauma? If yes, describe that episode.
h.	When did that trauma or accident occur?
i.	Was the arrival of pain gradual or sudden?
j.	Was there a change in lifestyle, such as a change in job/work setting/exercise/sport/life prior to the event?

2. ✎ __ Take an inventory of your life to understand potential sources of your pain. Simply circle "**Yes**" or "**No**" below and list your injury history.

3. ✎ __ Do you have older (more than three months) injuries/surgeries/conditions from childhood to the present day, regardless of whether you think they may be connected to your current pain? **Yes/No**

    If **Yes**, list them below. Be specific, i.e. left kneecap dislocation in 1995, multiple right shoulder strains in 2005, etc.) Put them in chronological order beginning with the oldest as #1 (expand this list as necessary):

1		6	
2		7	
3		8	
4		9	
5		10	

4. ✎. __ Put an "X" to the left of the number after which you began experiencing the pain you identified in Question #1. For instance, if you have seven older problems and your pain began after the occurrence of the 4th problem, you would put an "X" by #4. This may indicate that problems prior to #4 may have contributed to your current pain. It may also indicate that problems from #4 through #7 may also be caused by those same issues. At this point, don't worry about the ramifications of your answers—it is likely that the truth will be revealed soon.

5. ✎. __ Do you experience anxiety, stress, depression or have you experienced emotional trauma? **Yes/No**

    If **Yes**, list those issues below. Be as specific as possible—it helps to see what your brain is processing (expand this list as necessary and provide as much detail as you like—this is private and for your eyes only). If possible, list the year these issues began. Begin with the oldest issue first:

1		6
2		7
3		8
4		9
5		10

6. ✎. __ Put an "X" to the left of the number after which you began experiencing pain which you identified in Question #1. Apply the same thinking to the question in #3 to this list as well. Are there any possible connections?

7. ✎. __ Do you experience food intolerances/allergies or believe there may be mold exposure or other internal stressors? **Yes/No**

    If **Yes**, list those issues below. Be as specific as possible (expand this list as necessary). If possible, list the year these issues began. Begin with the oldest issue first:

1		6
2		7
3		8
4		9
5		10

Put an "X" to the left of the number after which you began experiencing the pain you identified in Question #1. Apply the same thinking to the question in #3 to this list as well. Are there any connections?

8.   ✎ __ Take a step back and objectively look at your three lists. Perhaps even show them to someone you trust—your medical practitioner, therapist, a close friend, or family member. Sometimes an objective eye will see things more clearly. Is there a pattern that seems to have emerged from these lists? **Yes/No**

9.   ✎ __ Finally, assign percentages to the three pillars of pain based on your lists and any feedback you have received. Only you can determine how to weigh your history. For instance, you may have sustained multiple musculoskeletal injuries when younger but suffered a significant emotional trauma, after which either these injuries began occurring or after which your pain began to emerge. In that case, you may give more weight to emotional trauma as a driver of your pain, even though those injuries may be factors too. You don't need to be 100% correct at this point, because you haven't tested your theories. Simply go with your history and your gut on these percentages at this point in time:

Musculoskeletal/Movement causes	%
Emotional/Psychological causes	%
Internal/Allergens/Mold causes	%

10. ✎ __ Based on Question #8, do you think there could be issues other than Musculoskeletal/Movement problems contributing to your pain (remember, it could be a small contribution, rather than 100%)? **Yes/No**

If you answered "**Yes**," then it may be worthwhile exploring these potential sources while also addressing musculoskeletal problems. But who should you turn to? In my experience, finding a therapist to help work through your psychological issues is extremely helpful—especially while solving musculoskeletal problems. Remember that the funnel works both ways—fixing the body soothes the mind and may help release long-held psychological tension just as soothing the mind can help the body release physical tension. In addition to therapists in your area, there are several good and affordable online mental health websites where you can work one-on-one with a therapist without leaving your home.

Regarding internal issues/allergens/molds etc., naturopathic doctors are a good source of help, especially if you have already been down the traditional medical route yet suspect there may be an environmental cause. These professionals are medically trained, test for problems outside the traditional medical scope of practice and understand how to address issues that turn up on these tests.

Functional medical practitioners can also be a good source for alternative testing and solutions, although few have undergone traditional medical training. They have a variety of backgrounds and beliefs they bring to their practice so, like any health or medical professional, be sure to do your homework before placing your trust in someone.

11.   ✎ ___ Develop a loose plan to move forward with whatever you have uncovered.

Based on the information above, in the next four weeks, I will (fill out all three steps):

1	
2	
3	

Take-Home Points

1.   There are three types of issues potentially creating most forms of pain: Musculoskeletal, Psychological, and/or Dietary.

2.   Listing events in chronological order can help expose hidden sources or connections to pain.

3.   Prioritizing and addressing those hidden sources can often be the key to unlocking tension and pain.

Chapter 20   Which Exercises Will Solve My Pain?

Congratulations! You now have a greater understanding of how chronic tension and pain are created in your body and you have completed several tests to specifically identify fundamental patterns behind your pain. You have also identified other potential sources of problems contributing to your tension and pain.

The big picture from this book is that we must reframe our ideas of pain from something that should be avoided to that of larger pain patterns your body is experiencing. You now have an idea of how to interpret and test these messages as well as begin correcting them.

Each time you perform some task or movement that is causing you pain, such as bending over, see it as an opportunity to understand what you have learned more deeply. The tools in this book will help you identify the problems associated with those movements in order to fix them. While a problem may have its roots in an accident/event which occurred years ago, it is still stressing your system now. Fix that problem today and your body will flourish once again, just as it was designed to.

In my clinical experience, pain reduces rapidly when problems causing pain are eliminated. This is so consistent and immediate that I can quickly work through several movement modifications and/or exercises in a single 30-minute session to find the pain culprits. This makes figuring out what helps and what hurts very simple, using what I call a Test/Retest strategy.

Test/Retest 📽

Because pain is an indication that something is wrong now, it should respond now to the removal or correction of that problem. Over the years I've devised a test/re-test strategy to quickly identify the most beneficial exercises or eliminate/modify those that aren't helpful. Here's how to use the Test/Retest strategy:

Step 1.

Test your pain by performing a certain movement or behavior that elicits *immediate* pain (refer to Question #1 from Chapter 19 to drill down into details). For example, if you sit down and cross your left ankle over your right knee and this immediately triggers your left sciatic pain, then this would become your test. Be sure to note the precise range of motion and pain level (0–10) associated with this movement. If the pain takes several seconds or a couple of minutes to emerge, then note the time or repetitions or distance. You want a clear test with consistent and measurable responses that appear relatively quickly.

Step 2.

Write down details of the movement, exercise, or behavior below that triggers your pain and your level of pain. Please be as specific as possible:

✎. __ Pain-producing behavior (include range of motion restrictions): _____

✎. __ Pain level (0–10) when performing that behavior: _____

✎. __ Other factors necessary to create pain (time, steps, repetitions, etc.): _____

Step 3.

Perform two sets of an exercise from Chapters 6–14 that you have discovered as identifying possible problems feeding your pain pattern. If you are using my digital home program, it would be an exercise from the *Pain Reduction* phase of that program or the *Somatics Audio Lessons* (also provided in this book). Alternatively, please feel free to use any exercise anyone has given you claiming it will solve your pain problem(s).

Step 4.

Immediately retest your original painful movement or behavior from #1 to see if that pain has reduced, if you can move further with less or no pain, if the pain takes longer to manifest, or if you simply seem to have to search for the pain a little more.

Was that exercise helpful in reducing your pain? **Yes/No** (circle one)

If "**Yes**" then you now know that exercise is important in solving your pain.

If "**No**" then that exercise either is less helpful or not helpful at all (assuming you did the exercise correctly).

If your pain actually increased after doing that exercise, then you know that exercise is likely the opposite of what you should be doing or that it contains elements that tap into your pain pattern. This exercise then can also become a test/retest behavior.

In all three scenarios, it is important to understand the "Why." Let us break these results down.

1. "**Yes**" that exercise reduced my pain. The next question is "Why?" Your body is trying to show you a solution. Does that solution align with any of the tests you have performed in this book? Does it fit into any of the three patterns of problems identified in this book (Extension, Flexion, Sidebending)? Think about it. Reread the pertinent chapters from this book to help you connect the dots.

2. "**No**" that exercise did not change my pain. Then you can probably check that off of your list of things to do today, provided that you performed the exercise correctly. It is a neutral exercise that does not teach you anything other than something you can do that has no effect on your pain.

3. "**That made my pain worse**." Once again, your body is trying to show you where the problem is. Try to break down that exercise into smaller parts—perhaps video yourself performing the exercise so you can more objectively critique it. Can you find a particular element that hurts? If a particular exercise can make your pain worse, then something should also make it better. Break down that movement or exercise into smaller pieces. Does *every* aspect of the exercise cause pain or is it just one small part of it? Which part is actually causing the pain? Does that part align with any of the tests you have performed in this book or any of the pain patterns? Think about it. Now experiment with modifying the part of that exercise you think is hurting you to align with the principles from this book. For instance, if you have discovered you have an Extension Problem, but you are arching your back to perform an exercise, such as the Butt Pump (Chapter 10), then that may be causing your pain rather than activating the butt muscles. Eliminate that arching on your next attempt. Is there less pain? Now you are working *with* your body to understand your pain patterns!

You can then apply this thinking to any exercise or solution. This may help you drill down more quickly on those exercises/habits/behaviors that actually help you and avoid those that hurt you. If there is a cluster of three exercises that help you, ask yourself "Why?" Do they all address the same type of muscle, joint or pattern of movement? Do they solve one of the three primary pain patterns you have identified in this book?

Systems thinking is the language your body uses to communicate with you. I hope that this book will help you decipher your lessons and that you will find them as fascinating as my patients and I have over the years.

Take-Home Points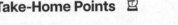

1. Chronic pain is a signal that something is wrong now and addressing that problem can create immediate changes in the level of pain.

2. Using a Test/Retest strategy is an efficient means of discovering which exercises help or hurt your efforts to resolve your pain.

3. Applying what you have learned from the Test/Retest strategy to understand your larger patterns of tension and pain will help you identify and correct problems throughout the day.

Chapter 21 Methods to Reduce Tension and Pain

Movement, fascia, and larger reflex patterns weave together to create chronic pain. The tests, confounding factors and strategies featured in Chapters 6–20 reveal the hidden mechanisms that often drive these patterns, as well as exercises or habit adjustments required to begin dismantling them. This chapter offers alternative methods that can also help to reduce tension associated with pain.

Meditation

Meditation calms the body and mind by focusing on breathing or awareness. This helps stimulate our rest and digest nervous system (PSNS) and reduce the fight or flight nervous system (SNS) which is associated with increased tension and pain (Chapter 3). There are many apps, podcasts and YouTube videos that teach meditation.

One study found that Zen meditation can even increase nitrite and nitrate serum concentrations in the blood.[54] These molecules are biomarkers of nitric oxide (NO) production helpful for reducing fascial tension (see **Laser Therapy** below).

A simple way to get started is to exhale for longer than you inhale. Sit or lie down comfortably. Inhale through your nose, then exhale a little longer through your mouth, for example breathe in for five seconds and exhale for eight seconds. Your mind will likely wander but simply bring it back to your breathing awareness. Sense areas of your body that are tense and try to relax them. Set a timer for three minutes and see how you feel afterwards. Practicing this technique, you might find that you almost immediately begin to feel more calm.

Surprisingly, there is little research to support that meditation has a significant impact on chronic pain.[55] While it may not have an empirically demonstrable direct relationship, in my experience meditation skills are involved in solving chronic tension and pain. Reducing chronic tension involves becoming more self-aware of subconscious habits, tension or mindsets that may be contributing to pain. From this standpoint, practice taking time to scan your thoughts and body and calming yourself using these simple meditation techniques. It will be time well spent.

Box Breathing

A variation of this is box breathing. Sitting or lying down comfortably, simply inhale, hold your breath briefly, exhale, hold your breath briefly, then repeat. You can visualize this technique as forming a box whereby the inhale is moving up the vertical face, the breath hold is the horizontal top surface, the exhale is moving down the other vertical face, and then finally the breath hold at the bottom is the flat surface of your box, resting on the ground (Figure 21.1).

Try to exhale for longer than your inhale to stimulate the PSNS which then shortens the breath hold at the bottom of the box (Figure 21.2).

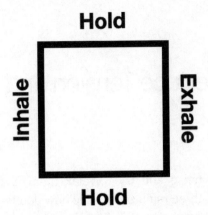

Figure 21.1. Box Breathing can be visualized as using your breath to form a square or rectangular pattern.

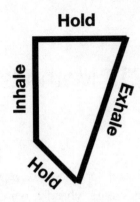

Figure 21.2. Box Breathing with a longer exhale shortens the breath hold at the bottom.

Box Breathing + Contraction 🎥

Now let's take this up a notch. This time, when you inhale, scrunch up your face as if you are in intense pain, are angry or as if you had just bitten into a really sour lemon. Hold this face and your breath at the top of the box, then slowly let those face muscles relax as you exhale. Feel different parts of your face releasing their tension. Try to time it so that your muscles relax at the same time that you have finished exhaling. Note how relaxed your face and head feel. Now take another breath while contracting your upper body muscles (bending your arms, making fists, hunching your shoulders, etc.) and your face as much as you can. Hold everything at the top of the box and then slowly release all those contracted muscles while exhaling. Rest and sense how your body now feels.

Are there some muscles that are more reluctant to relax? Think about those and see if you can change that on your next attempt. Continue this for a couple more times, trying to find as many muscles as you can to contract and then slowly release each one during the exhale. Feel free to lie down and explore contracting other areas of your body while box breathing as well. Then rest and assess.

Laugh It Off!

When was the last time you really laughed? Yes, there is a thing called Laughter Therapy and it has even been found to reduce emotional stress and anxiety.[56] Personally, nothing helps me break out of my own anxiety or stress better than a good laugh. The bigger the laugh, the more release I feel. There are many ways to have a good laugh: YouTube videos, Netflix or Amazon Prime comedy shows (I'm a big fan of Jim Gaffigan and John Mulaney), live comedy, TV programs, or just simply reading corny Dad jokes on the internet. I now regularly listen to funny podcasts to keep my mood up and tension levels down, especially when doing chores around the house I hate doing. My two favorites are *Conan O'Brien Needs a Friend* and *Smartless*.

Laser Therapy

Laser therapy is one of the few modalities I have found that can produce rapid, meaningful change to tension and pain. There are different classes of laser that correspond to their wattage. In my clinic, I had a Class 4 therapeutic laser (not to be confused with a hot or cold laser—which I think are misnomers). At the time of writing, a Class 4 laser was the most powerful available. I was often amazed at its ability to quickly restore range of motion and reduce pain. This made it very popular at my clinic. While laser research touts increasing mitochondrial output (**mitochondria** are little energy factories in cells), the near instantaneous increase in range of motion and decrease in pain, in my mind, could not be attributable to that.

In my opinion, these results could only be explained by addressing fascial restrictions. It turns out that one of the biproducts of laser treatment is that it increases the body's local production of NO (nitric oxide).[57] Nitric oxide is a gas synthesized in the body that is integral to smooth muscle contraction, neurotransmission, and organ inflammation modulation.[58] Remember in Chapter 3 we covered that fascia is invested with smooth muscle? There may be indications that myofibroblasts relax in the presence of NO.[59,60] To me this explains the mechanism of laser treatment in terms of rapidly restoring function. Perhaps trying a few sessions of Class 4 laser therapy with a local healthcare practitioner might help you see improved results.

Therapeutic Pools

The buoyancy provided by water can help unload painful joints and tissues, allowing more freedom of movement. Your brain has developed compensation patterns based on your weight-bearing strategies in response to ground-reaction forces. Reducing these forces seems to allow many of you to retrain movements out of habitual patterns more easily.

For this reason, therapeutic pools can often be the perfect place to begin when climbing out of a chronic pain condition. Many towns have recreational centers or retirement communities with therapeutic pools that may even be heated—talk about relaxing! Classes here can be deeply rewarding. You will also have the opportunity to make new friends. Just be sure to approach the instructor first so they are aware of your condition and intentions. They can then help you modify exercises as necessary. If you want to work alone, there are videos on YouTube of pool exercises you can try. I would be careful to keep it simple and short during your first few visits until you understand how your body responds. You can always add on from there.

Hanna Somatics

Hanna Somatics involves applying the neurological, fascial, and musculoskeletal information from this book to the patterns of tension corresponding to the three elemental patterns of dysfunction discovered by Dr. Shirley Sahrmann, Thomas Myers, and Dr. Thomas Hanna.

Moving freely and without tension reduces wear and tear on the body as well as emotional strain. In my clinical experience, eliminating tension helps clear the slate so that you can see where the specific causes of that tension are coming from. When the body is more relaxed, it becomes easier to spot those activities that cause it to feel tense again. Until we break the tension/pain cycle, we feel completely unable to beat it. Breaking this cycle, even briefly, will reassure you that there is a path to unraveling these pain patterns and will show you where to begin.

In my experience, the principles of Hanna Somatics have been invaluable to penetrate this tension pattern problem. We must incorporate the brain using specific neurological pathways described earlier, to reset muscle spindles monitoring length and tension. Resetting these spindles, especially in the larger patterns of movement identified by these three researchers, is a game-changer for most of you caught in a tension/pain cycle.

It is much easier than you think. In fact, if you tried the meditation exercise I described earlier (Box Breathing + Contraction), where I asked you to contract your upper body muscles and sync that with your breathing, all you did was apply all that complicated neuroscience. You contracted your muscles voluntarily (motor cortex and cerebellar involvement via corticospinal tract) then slowly released those contracted muscles (controlled eccentric contraction while lengthening and resetting the muscle spindles) which were mediated along the spinocerebellar, DCML, and corticospinal tracts, in coordination with your motor and sensory cortices. At the same time, while lengthening your exhale, you stimulated your PSNS (rest and digest nervous system), which inhibited your SNS (fight or flight nervous system).

So, hopefully, you now have a greater appreciation for what is going on behind the scenes in order to create movement, and you feel much more relaxed, physically and mentally, after that simple exercise. However, that was a non-specific application of these ideas—just imagine what would happen if that intention was directed along the three patterns of problems behind almost all pain.

The most common reaction to the effects of Hanna Somatics is one of surprise. Most of you who are caught in a chronic tension pattern cycle have a hard time believing such simple exercises can have a powerful effect on your pain. This is also because you have been living with tension and pain for so long that you have forgotten how it feels to move freely (SMA). This is why I have included three audio Hanna Somatics movement lessons, each designed to address a different pattern of tension found in the body, that can be accessed together with the videos of tests and exercises from this book.

Lesson 1 addresses tension along the Extension Problem pattern (also the back line of fascia or the Landau Reflex pattern) which you tested in Chapter 6. Most of you with back or sciatic pain have this problem as one of your patterns.

Lesson 3 addresses tension along the Sidebending Problem pattern (also the lateral/spiral lines of fascia or the Withdrawal/Crossed Extensor Reflex pattern) which you tested in Chapter 7. As you might imagine, those of you with unilateral back pain, sciatic pain, or SI joint pain typically have the Sidebending Problem as one of your patterns. Most of you suffering from chronic pain have both of these patterns.

Lesson 8 is quite unusual and addresses walking—the common behavior functionally linking all lower body or back patterns of tension and pain.

To access your free Hanna Somatics lessons and other tests and exercises from this book, visit: www.rickolderman.com, then select the "Books" tab and scroll down to find the *Pain Patterns* book videos. Type in the code: PainPatterns

Whether the source of your pain is musculo-skeletal, emotional, or dietary, all three pillars lead most of you to similar patterns of tension that create pain—Extension, Flexion, and/or Sidebending Problems. My hope is that you now realize most of you should begin by understanding what patterns are creating your pain and why. The Hanna Somatics lessons provided with this book are a good place to begin unraveling the tension that holds these patterns together.

Some of you only need Hanna Somatics lessons to keep your pain at bay. However, there are also tight or weak muscles and poor movement habits, like walking, bending, and sitting that perpetuate pain. You can use the Test/Retest strategy from Chapter 20 to help you identify which exercises are helpful or harmful when working toward your goals.

I wish you all the best in your search for solutions and I hope that this book has expanded your awareness of why you are experiencing pain and how you can move forward. Reframing your pain as patterns of problems that are occurring in the present will help you successfully solve the problems causing your pain.

Take-Home Points

1. There are many methods to reduce tension and pain.

2. Hanna Somatics has become a powerful tool in my clinical experience to reduce patterns of tension and pain and is a good place to begin when exploring tension reduction techniques.

Acknowledgements

I would like to thank Dr. Shirley Sahrmann, Thomas Myers, and Dr. Thomas Hanna for their passion, research, and dedication to helping people and other therapists solve difficult pain problems.

Thank you also to my brother, Russ, who helped make this book more readable through his many edits.

Thank you also to my medical illustrators: Martin Huber, Meghan Lewis and Bence Berszán Árus, who created unique images to portray key concepts in this book.

Finally, I would like to thank my patients, past and future, for their willingness to consider and explore new ideas about why they have pain and how to solve it.

Thank you to Urška Charney for making this book more readable through her skill in design and layout.

Recommended Reading

Hanna, Thomas. *Somatics: Reawakening The Mind's Control Of Movement, Flexibility, And Health*. Da Capo Press, 2004.

Myers, Thomas W. *Anatomy Trains: Myofascial Meridians for Manual Therapists & Movement Practitioners*, 4th ed, Elsevier, 2021.

Schleip, Robert; Stecco, Carla; Driscoll, Mark; Huijing, Peter A. *Fascia: The Tensional Network of the Human Body*, 2nd ed, Elsevier, 2022.

Sahrmann, Shirley A. *Diagnosis and Treatment of Movement Impairment Syndromes*. Mosby, 2001.

Index

Endnotes

1   Heick, J. Lazaro, RT (2023, Elsevier) *Goodman and Snyder's Differential Diagnosis for Physical Therapists: Screening for Referral,* 7th Edition.

2   Raja SN, Carr DB, Cohen M, Finnerup NB, Flor H, Gibson S, Keefe FJ, Mogil JS, Ringkamp M, Sluka KA, Song XJ, Stevens B, Sullivan MD, Tutelman PR, Ushida T, Vader K. The revised International Association for the Study of Pain definition of pain: concepts, challenges, and compromises. *Pain.* 2020 Sep 1;161(9):1976-1982.

3   Brinjikji W, Luetmer PH, Comstock B, Bresnahan BW, Chen LE, Deyo RA, Halabi S, Turner JA, Avins AL, James K, Wald JT, Kallmes DF, Jarvik JG. Systematic literature review of imaging features of spinal degeneration in asymptomatic populations. *AJNR Am J Neuroradiol.* 2015 Apr;36(4):811-6.

4   Sahrmann, S.A. (2002, Mosby) *Diagnosis and Treatment of Movement Impairment Syndromes.* St. Louis, MO.3 - 4

5   Sahrmann, S.A. (2002, Mosby) Diagnosis and Treatment of Movement Impairment Syndromes. St. Louis, MO: 51 - 120

6   Sahrmann, S.A. (2002, Mosby) *Diagnosis and Treatment of Movement Impairment Syndromes.* St. Louis, MO: 10 - 11

7   Sahin M. S., Ergün A., Aslan A. (2015). The relationship between osteoarthritis of the lumbar facet joints and lumbosacropelvic morphology. Spine 40, E1058–E1062.

8   Müller A, Rockenfeller R, Damm N, Kosterhon M, Kantelhardt SR, Aiyangar AK, Gruber K. Load Distribution in the Lumbar Spine During Modeled Compression Depends on Lordosis. *Front Bioeng Biotechnol.* 2021 Jun 10;9:661258.

9   Chun S. W., Lim C. Y., Kim K., Hwang J., Chung S. G. (2017). The relationships between low back pain and lumbar lordosis: A systematic review and meta-analysis. *The Spine Journal* 17, 1180–1191.

10 Müller A, Rockenfeller R, Damm N, Kosterhon M, Kantelhardt SR, Aiyangar AK, Gruber K. Load Distribution in the Lumbar Spine During Modeled Compression Depends on Lordosis. *Front Bioeng Biotechnol.* 2021 Jun 10;9:661258

11 Dydyk AM, Ngnitewe Massa R, Mesfin FB. Disc Herniation. [Updated 2023 Jan 16]. In: StatPearls [Internet]. Treasure Island (FL): StatPearls Publishing; 2024 Jan-

12 FN Fascia: The Tensional Network of the Human Body, 2nd edition, Elsevier, 2022, 157

13 FN Anatomy Trains: Myofascial Meridians for Manual and Movement Therapists, Elsevier, 2021, 1

14 FN Anatomy Trains: Myofascial Meridians for Manual and Movement Therapists, Elsevier, 2021, 147

15 FN Anatomy Trains: Myofascial Meridians for Manual and Movement Therapists, Elsevier, 2021, 148

16 Schleip, Robert, "Fascial plasticity—A new neurobiological explanation: Part 1," *Journal of Bodywork and Movement Therapies, Jan 2003,* 7 (2), 104-16.

17 Schleip R, Gabbiani G, Wilke J, Naylor I, Hinz B, Zorn A, Jäger H, Breul R, Schreiner S, Klingler W. Fascia Is Able to Actively Contract and May Thereby Influence Musculoskeletal Dynamics: A Histochemical and Mechanographic Investigation. *Front Physiol.* 2019 Apr 2;10:336.

18 Schleip, Robert; Stecco, Carla; Driscoll, Mark; Hiding, Peter. Fascia: The Tensional Network of the Human Body, 2nd ed. pgs. 180-183. Elsevier, 2022.

19 Tai Y, Woods EL, Dally J, Kong D, Steadman R, Moseley R, Midgley AC. Myofibroblasts: Function, Formation, and Scope of Molecular Therapies for Skin Fibrosis. *Biomolecules.* 2021 Jul 23;11(8):1095.

20 Näther P, Kersten JF, Kaden I, Irga K, Nienhaus A. Distribution Patterns of Degeneration of the Lumbar Spine in a Cohort of 200 Patients with an Indication for Lumbar MRI. Int J Environ Res Public Health. 2022 Mar 21;19(6):3721.21 Brown RA, Sethi KK, Gwanmesia I, Raemdonck D, Eastwood M, Mudera V. Enhanced fibroblast contraction of 3D collagen lattices and

integrin expression by TGF-beta1 and -beta3: mechanoregulatory growth factors? *Exp Cell Res.* 2002 Apr 1;274(2):310-22.

22 Schleip R, Gabbiani G, Wilke J, Naylor I, Hinz B, Zorn A, Jäger H, Breul R, Schreiner S, Klingler W. Fascia Is Able to Actively Contract and May Thereby Influence Musculoskeletal Dynamics: A Histochemical and Mechanographic Investigation. *Front Physiol.* 2019 Apr 2;10:336.

23 Bhowmick, S., Singh, A., Flavell, R.A., Clark, R.B., O'Rourke, J., & Cone, R.E. (2009). The sympathetic nervous system modulates CD4(+)FoxP3(+) regulatory T cells via a TGF-beta-dependent mechanism. *J Leukoc Biol, 86*(6), 1275–1283.

24 Tomasek, J.J, Gabbiani, G., Hinz, B., Chaponnier, C., & Brown, R.A. (2002). Myofibroblasts and mechano-reg- ulation of connective tissue remodeling. *Nat Rev Mol Cell Biol, 3*, 349-363.

25 Liao MH, Liu SS, Peng IC, Tsai FJ, Huang HH. The stimulatory effects of alpha1-adrenergic receptors on TGF-beta1, IGF-1 and hyaluronan production in human skin fibroblasts. *Cell Tissue Res.* 2014 Sep;357(3):681-93.

26 Dalton, Erik, et al., *Dynamic body: Exploring form, expanding function* (Freedom from Pain Institute, 2011), 153–54.

27 Schleip R, Gabbiani G, Wilke J, Naylor I, Hinz B, Zorn A, Jäger H, Breul R, Schreiner S, Klingler W. Fascia Is Able to Actively Contract and May Thereby Influence Musculoskeletal Dynamics: A Histochemical and Mechanographic Investigation. Front Physiol. 2019 Apr 2;10:336.

28 Tsao, Henry, Mary P. Galea, and Paul W. Hodges. "Driving plasticity in the motor cortex in recurrent low back pain." *European journal of pain* 14.8 (2010): 832-839.

29 Al-Chalabi, M, Reddy V, Alsalman I. Neuroanatomy, Posterior Column (Dorsal Column) [Updated 2023 Apr 8]. In: StatPearls [Internet]. Treasure Island (FL): StatPearls Publishing; 2023 Jan-.

30 Macefield, VG; Knellwolf, TP (1 August 2018). "Functional properties of human muscle spindles." *Journal of Neurophysiology.* 120 (2): 452–467.

31 Fan C, Pirri C, Fede C, Guidolin D, Biz C, Petrelli L, Porzionato A, Macchi V, De Caro R, Stecco C. Age-Related Alterations of Hyaluronan and Collagen in Extracellular Matrix of the Muscle Spindles. J Clin Med. 2021 Dec 24;11(1):86.

32 Ovalle WK, Dow PR, Nahirney PC. Structure, distribution and innervation of muscle spindles in avian fast and slow skeletal muscle. J Anat. 1999 Apr;194 (Pt 3)(Pt 3):381-94

33 Alfvén G, Grillner S, Andersson E. Children with chronic stress-induced recurrent muscle pain have enhanced startle reaction. *Eur J Pain.* 2017 Oct;21(9):1561-1570.

34 Flor H, Turk DC, Birbaumer N. Assessment of stress-related psychophysiological reactions in chronic back pain patients. *Journal of Consulting and Clinical Psychology.* 1985;53(3):354–364.

35 Fascia: The Tensional Network of the Human Body, Elsevier, 2022, 157-8.

36 Sahrmann, S.A. (2002, Mosby) Diagnosis and Treatment of Movement Impairment Syndromes. St. Louis, MO. 3

37 Sahrmann, S.A. (2002, Mosby) Diagnosis and Treatment of Movement Impairment Syndromes. St. Louis, MO. 13

38 Meakin LB, Galea GL, Sugiyama T, Lanyon LE, Price JS. 2014. Age-related impairment of bones' adaptive response to loading in mice is associated with sex-related deficiencies in osteoblasts but no change in osteocytes. Journal of Bone and Mineral Research 29:1859–1871.

39 Hitomi Nakamura, Kazuhiro Aoki, Wataru Masuda, Neil Alles, Kenichi Nagano, Hidefumi Fukushima, Kenji Osawa, Hisataka Yasuda, Ichiro Nakamura, Yuko Mikuni␡Takagaki, Keiichi Ohya, Kenshi Maki, Eijiro Jimi, Disruption of NF-κB1 prevents bone loss caused by mechanical unloading, Journal of Bone and Mineral Research, Volume 28, Issue 6, 1 June 2013, Pages 1457–1467.

40 Zöllner AM, Pok JM, McWalter EJ, Gold GE, Kuhl E. On high heels and short muscles: a multiscale model for sarcomere loss in the gastrocnemius muscle. J Theor Biol. 2015 Jan 21;365:301-10. doi: 10.1016/j.jtbi.2014.10.036. Epub 2014 Nov 7

41 Wuertz-Kozak K, Roszkowski M, Cambria E, Block A, Kuhn GA, Abele T, Hitzl W, Drießlein D, Müller R, Rapp MA, Mansuy IM, Peters EMJ, Wippert PM. Effects of Early Life Stress on Bone Homeostasis in Mice and Humans. Int J Mol Sci. 2020 Sep 10;21(18):6634

42 Schleip. Fascia: The Tensional Network of the Human Body, 2nd ed. Elsevier, 2022. pg. 336-7

43 Sutton KM, Bullock JM. Anterior cruciate ligament rupture: differences between males and females. *J Am Acad Orthop Surg*. 2013 Jan;21(1):41-50.

44 Kumar A, Pramanik J, Goyal N, Chauhan D, Sivamaruthi BS, Prajapati BG, Chaiyasut C. Gut *Microbiota in Anxiety and Depression: Unveiling the Relationships and Management Options. Pharmaceuticals* (Basel). 2023 Apr 9;16(4):565.

45 Chin Fatt, C.R., Asbury, S., Jha, M.K. et al. Leveraging the microbiome to understand clinical heterogeneity in depression: findings from the T-RAD study. *Transl Psychiatry 13*, 139 (2023).

46 Mahroum N, Seida R, Shoenfeld Y. Triggers and regulation: the gut microbiome in rheumatoid arthritis. *Expert Rev Clin Immunol*. 2023 Jul-Dec;19(12):1449-1456 and Breban M. Gut microbiota and inflammatory joint diseases. *Joint Bone Spine*. 2016 Dec;83(6):645-649.

47 Breban M. Gut microbiota and inflammatory joint diseases. *Joint Bone Spine*. 2016 Dec;83(6):645-649.

48 Chin RL, Sander HW, Brannagan TH, et al. Celiac neuropathy. *Neurology*. 2003;60:1581-5.

49 Cicarelli G, Della Rocca G, Amboni M, et al. Clinical and neurological abnormalities in adult celiac disease. *Neurol Sci*. 2003;24:311-7.

50 Cooke W, Smith W. Neurological disorders associated with adult celiac disease. *Brain*. 1966;89:683-722.

51 Schneider S.M. Al-Jaouni R. Filippi J. Wiroth J.B. Zeanandin G. Arab K. et al. Sarcopenia is prevalent in patients with Crohn's disease in clinical remission *Inflamm Bowel Dis* 14 2008 1562-1568

52 Wiroth J.B. Filippi J. Schneider S.M. Al-Jaouni R. Horvais N. Gavarry O. et al. Muscle performance in patients with Crohn's disease in clinical remission *Inflamm Bowel Dis* 11 2005 296-303.

53 Geerling B.J. Badart-Smook A. Stockbrugger R.W. Brummer R.J. Comprehensive nutritional status in patients with long-standing Crohn disease currently in remission *Am J Clin Nutr* 67 1998 919-926.

54 Kim DH, Moon YS, Kim HS, Jung JS, Park HM, Suh HW, Kim YH, Song DK. Effect of Zen Meditation on serum nitric oxide activity and lipid peroxidation. *Prog Neuropsychopharmacol Biol Psychiatry*. 2005 Feb;29(2):327-31.

55 Lara Hilton, Susanne Hempel, Brett A. Ewing, Eric Apaydin, Lea Xenakis, Sydne Newberry, Ben Colaiaco, Alicia Ruelaz Maher, Roberta M. Shanman, Melony E. Sorbero, Margaret A. Maglione, Mindfulness Meditation for Chronic Pain: Systematic Review and Meta-analysis, *Annals of Behavioral Medicine*, Volume 51, Issue 2, April 2017, Pages 199–213.

56 Hatzipapas I, Visser MJ, Janse van Rensburg E. Laughter therapy as an intervention to promote psychological well-being of volunteer community care workers working with HIV-affected families. *SAHARA J*. 2017 Dec;14(1):202-212.

57 Mitchell UH, Mack GL. Low-level laser treatment with near-infrared light increases venous nitric oxide levels acutely: a single-blind, randomized clinical trial of efficacy. *Am J Phys Med Rehabil*. 2013 Feb;92(2):151-6.

58 Robbins RA, Grisham MB. Nitric oxide. *Int J Biochem Cell Biol*. 1997 Jun;29(6):857-60.

59 Hoppe, K., et al. «Contractile elements in muscular fascial tissue–implications for in-vitro contracture testing for malignant hyperthermia." *Anaesthesia* 69.9 (2014): 1002-1008.

60 Schleip, Robert, W. Klingler, and F. Lehmann-Horn. "Fascia is able to contract in a smooth muscle-like manner and thereby influence musculoskeletal mechanics." *Journal of Biomechanics* 39 (2006): S488.

About the Author

Rick Olderman graduated from Krannert School of Physical Therapy at the University of Indianapolis in 1996. He lives in Denver, CO with his wife and two children. Rick enjoys traveling, gardening, fishing, speaking, trail running and camping.

Visit www.rickolderman.com and then "Fixing You Programs" to learn more about his digital home programs to solve pain. Enter the discount code: PainPatterns to receive 25% off your order.

Subscribe to Rick's YouTube channel to watch his latest videos that help people understand and solve their pain.

Rick's books are available on Amazon and include:

Fixing You: Back Pain & Sciatica
Fixing You: Neck Pain & Headaches
Fixing You: Hip & Knee Pain
Fixing You: Foot & Ankle Pain
Fixing You: Back Pain During Pregnancy
Solving the Pain Puzzle: Cases from 25 Years as a Physical Therapist
Top 3 Fix: Bob & Brad's (and Rick's) 3 Most Effective Exercises to Solve Pain from Headaches to Plantar Fasciitis (co-written with Bob Schrupp PT)

Health or wellness practitioners can learn Rick's methods in his CEU course at www.rickolderman.com then click "Practitioner Course."

Made in the USA
Thornton, CO
03/08/25 16:41:24

e9fbf692-f6ea-4cd1-aea9-f32dc9f7ffd2R01